Holistic
Aromatherapy

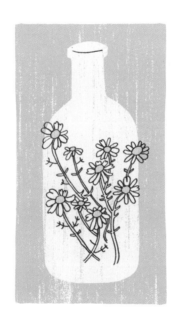

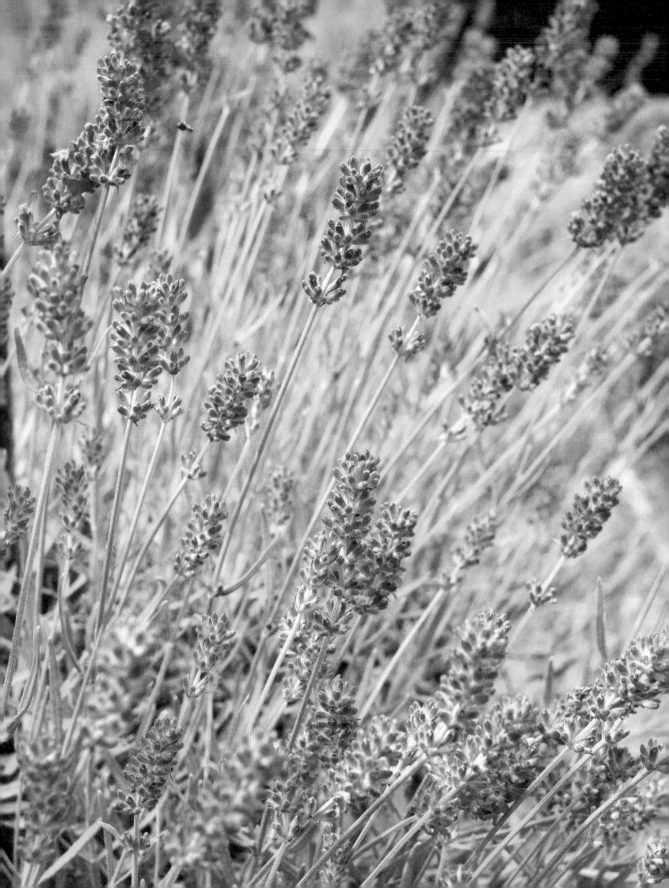

Holistic Aromatherapy

PRACTICAL SELF-HEALING WITH ESSENTIAL OILS

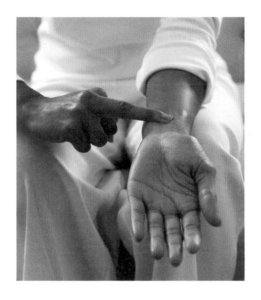

Marc J. Gian
L. Ac, LMT

CICO BOOKS
LONDON NEW YORK

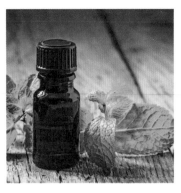

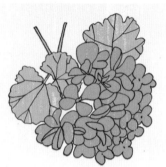

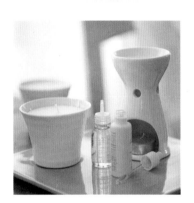

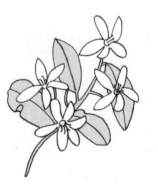

For my family

Published in 2017 by CICO Books
An imprint of Ryland Peters & Small Ltd
20–21 Jockey's Fields   341 E 116th St
London WC1R 4BW   New York, NY 10029

www.rylandpeters.com

10 9 8 7 6 5 4 3 2 1

A CIP catalog record for this book is available from the Library of
Congress and the British Library.

ISBN: 978-1-78249-441-6

Printed in China

Editor: Clare Churly
Designer: Emily Breen
Illustrators: Rosie Scott, Stephen Dew, and Cathy Brear

Commissioning editor: Kristine Pidkameny
Senior editor: Carmel Edmonds
Art director: Sally Powell
Production controller: Mai-Ling Collyer
Publishing manager: Penny Craig
Publisher: Cindy Richards

Safety note: Please note that while the descriptions of essential
oils and blends refer to healing benefits, they are not intended to
replace diagnosis of illness or ailments, or healing or medicine.
Always consult your doctor or other health professional in the
case of illness. Neither the author nor the publisher can be held
responsible for any claim arising out of the general information
and blends provided in this book.

Contents

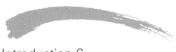

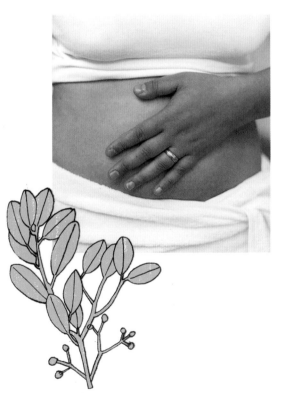

Introduction

Aromatherapy is the use of essential oils for healing and balancing the mind and body. It is through inhaling scents that healing occurs. It has become a popular form of treatment in recent years as people look for more natural ways to take control of their health. Essential oils are easily accessible and have proven to be very useful for personal health care. Some of the benefits of essential oils include relief from common colds and decreasing muscular pain.

Chinese medicine is a 3,000-year-old method of treating and preventing disease and calming the mind and emotions. It can provide the novice user of essential oils with an ancient but verified way to comprehend aromatherapy and enhance its healing benefits. Combining the foundations of Chinese medicine with aromatherapy creates a powerful synergy to bring balance to the mind and body. Both therapies have the ability to simultaneously treat the mind and the body and begin to connect us to the deepest, truest nature of our being.

Essential oils come from plants from all over the world: peppermint from Washington State, USA; Roman and German chamomile from the United Kingdom; lavender from France; bergamot from Italy; ravensara and ylang-ylang from Madagascar, tea tree and eucalyptus from Australia; to name but a few. Each oil has its own unique personality, or, in terms of Chinese medicine, its own spirit. The beauty of using essential oils based on Chinese medicine is that each oil correlates to specific acupressure points (see page 16), and applying oils to these points magnifies the healing.

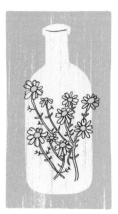 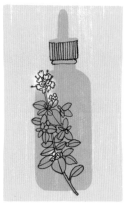 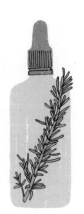 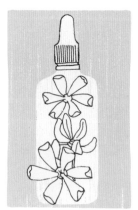 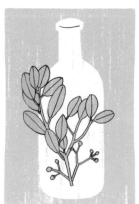

Over the past ten years or so there has been a steady increase and fascination with the use of essential oils and aroma to increase the clinical effectiveness of Chinese medicine and induce physical and emotional changes. Chinese medicine's practical applications—acupuncture, massage (tui na and acupressure), Chinese herbs, dietary therapy, qigong, and tai chi—take years to master. However, a novice can use the basics of massage with aromatherapy safely and effectively.

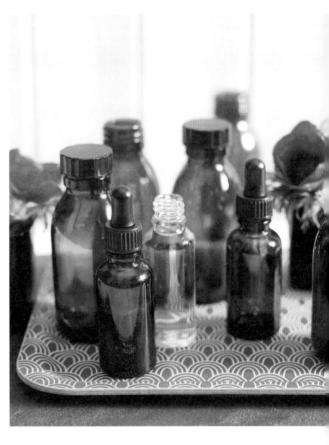

Chinese medicine aims to look at the whole person—not just the symptom or the body part—including the entire physical body, emotional tendencies, habits, and external environment. Likewise, exploring the source, physical features, habitat, and, of course, scent of a plant used to make an essential oil can lead to an understanding of the oil's unique functions and practical applications.

Chinese medicine views the body as a microcosm of the macrocosm—in other words, a part that contains a whole. Our body is a vessel that encompasses our history and present influence. This holds true in nature as well and can be seen in the plants and trees from which essential oils are derived. Plants often will take on the energy, or Qi (see page 12), of their natural habitat, and they will actually balance out their terrain. Rosemary, for instance, natively grows near the sea to help balance out the damp environment. In fact, one of the major functions of this oil is to transform Dampness (see page 39) and heaviness in the mind and body. Lavender is another good example of this principle. Lavender grows at high altitudes, and its oil is effective for treating the upper aspect of our bodies. Lavender is especially good for circulating Qi in the chest and relaxing the heart.

Do you want the tools to ignite a better physical, mental, and spiritual state of being? If your answer is "yes," then prepare for a journey into the healing world of essential oils and aromatherapy.

PART 1

THE

HEALING CONNECTION OF AROMATHERAPY AND CHINESE MEDICINE

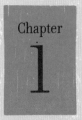

The Basics of Chinese Medicine

In order to understand the use of essential oils based on Traditional Chinese Medicine (TCM) you will need to become acquainted with the basics of TCM physiology and some of the most common terms used in Chinese medicine. Although there is no need to delve in depth into these principles, it is important to learn about the fundamental concepts of Yin and Yang, Qi, Blood, meridians and acupressure points, Jing, and the Shen. It is my hope that you will use these concepts not only to help you understand essential oils and Chinese medicine but also, more importantly, to develop a more holistic approach to contemplating and living a meaningful life.

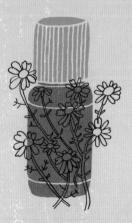

Yin and Yang

The concept of Yin and Yang is fundamental in Chinese medicine, and it is used to categorize everything in the universe. Yin and Yang are opposite forces by nature, yet neither can exist without the other. The two opposites make up a whole. They are contradictory yet inseparable, with Yin generally symbolizing darkness and Yang generally encompassing brightness. The sun and moon, day and night, and male and female are all clear examples of this theory.

Looking at the Yin and Yang symbol, you can see that there is a bit of Yin in Yang and bit of Yang in Yin. This highlights their interdependency and demonstrates that nothing is truly separate. For instance, during the daily cycle of the sun and moon, prime Yang is at 12 p.m. and as the day progresses it will eventually transform into prime Yin at 12 a.m.

When it comes to the human body, the back and spine are Yang in nature. These body parts are harder and more protected than the soft and vulnerable abdominal side, which is typically more Yin. The top of the head is also Yang, with the hardness of the skull as a protector, while the soft soles of the feet are Yin.

Essential oils can also be classified according to Yin or Yang. Oils made from leaves, such as rosemary and cinnamon leaf, are more Yang, while oils made from roots and resins, such as vetiver and myrrh, are more Yin.

THE FIVE KEY PRINCIPLES OF YIN AND YANG

1 Yin and Yang can be used to categorize all phenomena.
2 Yin and Yang are opposites.
3 Yin and Yang are divisible.
4 Yin and Yang are interdependent upon one another (you cannot have one without the other).
5 Yin and Yang balance and counterbalance one another.

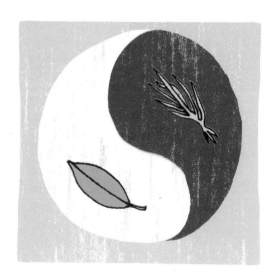

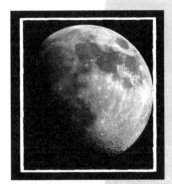

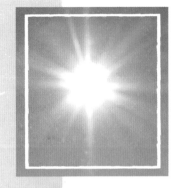

The Characteristics of Yin and Yang

YIN	YANG
Earth	Heaven
Cold	Hot
Moon	Sun
Winter	Summer
Night	Day
Receiving	Giving
Soft	Hard
Dark	Bright
Feminine	Masculine
Passive	Active
Water	Fire
Rest	Responsiveness
Interior	Exterior
Slow	Rapid
Blood	Qi
Front	Back
Downward	Upward
Front of body	Back of body
Feet	Head
Underside (palm side) of arm	Top side of arm
Lower body	Upper body

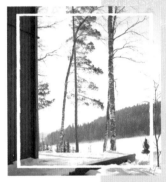

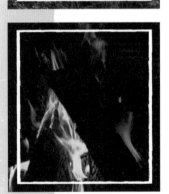

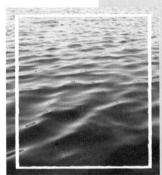

Yin and Yang are opposite forces by nature, yet neither can exist without the other.

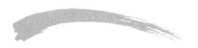

Qi

Qi is the electric, active nature of our power. The word "Qi" is commonly (and incompletely) translated as "life force." Qi is the exchange that fuels our reach into this world. It supports our bodily functions, physical activity, and mental activity. Qi is a concept that is difficult to define, and it is better understood by comprehending its functions. The four basic functions of Qi are moving or activating, warming, holding, and defending.

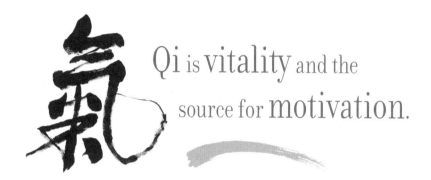

Qi is vitality and the source for motivation.

MOVING OR ACTIVATING

Qi is considered Yang because it is responsible for movement and activation, including digestion and growth. In other words, Qi is vitality and the source for motivation. In a healthy individual, Qi moves through the meridians (see page 16) and supports the building of Blood (see page 15).

Imbalance occurs when Qi is stuck (also known as Qi stagnation). The general symptoms of Qi stagnation include constipation, acid regurgitation, lack of flexibility, muscular pain, edema, headaches, depression, irritability, and frustration. The treatment strategy for Qi stagnation is to promote the movement of Qi. There are many oils that have the ability to relieve the different symptoms of Qi stagnation. For example, lemongrass is one of the best oils to use for hip pain that may or may not radiate down the Gall Bladder and Urinary Bladder meridians (the back of the legs). Inhaling the aroma of lavender or applying the essential oil to certain acupressure points will help to alleviate frustration and irritability, and it will also promote the movement of Liver Qi.

An insufficient quantity of Qi in the body will lead to a Qi deficiency or a lack of vitality. Major symptoms of Qi deficiency are frequent common colds, lethargy, muscle weakness, spontaneous sweating, loose stools, low libido, lower back pain, dizziness, a pale face, dislike of speaking, and low appetite. The treatment strategy for these symptoms is to tonify (strengthen and build) the Qi. The organ or meridian that is deficient in Qi will guide us to the correct oil. For example, if the Lungs are deficient in Qi, we can use ravensara to tonify the Lungs. If the Kidneys are deficient, especially with the symptoms of lower back pain, we can use Scots pine to stimulate Kidney Qi and bring relief to the pain.

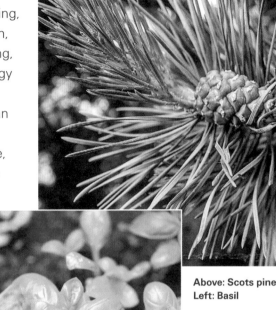

Above: Scots pine
Left: Basil

WARMING

Warming is another function of Qi. Warmth is imperative for the proper functioning of the organs and meridians. An adequate quantity of Qi and the warming function of the Kidneys supports the Stomach and Spleen in transforming and transporting postnatal Qi (see page 24) into Blood. Often, when there is not enough warmth in the body, we have the symptoms of Qi vacuity—a Qi deficiency when there is not enough Qi in the body to maintain the health of the body.

Spleen Qi deficiency is a common deficiency. Major symptoms include fatigue, muscle weakness, and loose stools. Specific essential oils that assist in tonifying the Spleen include rosemary, fennel, and basil.

HOLDING

Qi is responsible for holding or containing the functions of the body. It is through this function that Qi retains the fluids in the body and restrains them from leaking. Common examples of the way that Qi holds or contains bodily fluids include Lung Qi controlling the elimination of sweat, Spleen Qi containing the blood within blood vessels, and Kidney Qi holding urine and semen. When Qi does not hold it is a form of Qi or Yang deficiency.

When Qi's ability to hold is impaired we may see such symptoms such as spontaneous sweating, easy bruising, frequent urination, and premature ejaculation. In cases where we need to uplift or raise the Qi, rosemary is the premier oil.

DEFENDING

Wei Qi (also known as defensive Qi) is considered to be our protective layer, which in TCM terms resides between our skin and muscles. However, extending beyond TCM terms, such as in energetic medicine, there is also a protective layer around the body that guards us from pathogens in the outside world. Frequent common colds, for instance, are a symptom of a weakness in Wei Qi. However, on a more holistic note, strengthening Wei Qi can help us to create boundaries and guard against unwanted influences, particularly those from personal relationships. Cypress is a good oil to support Wei Qi.

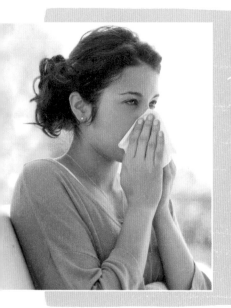

Exterior Conditions

Exterior conditions are those that affect the Wei level (the most external Qi of the body), such as the common cold and skin and muscle ailments.

- Releasing the Exterior is a common treatment strategy that is used when treating a common cold (Wind-Heat or Wind-Cold in TCM terms).
- Stabilizing the Exterior is a treatment strategy to make strong, impenetrable boundaries that are not vulnerable to external pathogenic influence.

Blood

Just like Yin and Yang, Blood and Qi are inseparable: Qi forms Blood, and Blood engenders Qi.

Blood is formed from postnatal Qi. The Stomach and Spleen turn food into postnatal Qi, which is then moved to the Lungs where the production of Blood is finalized, and then the Heart circulates the Blood throughout the body to provide nourishment.

Since things we experience can enter through the Wei level and move to the Ying level (see page 30), our experiences can also play a role in the transformation of Qi into Blood. Appreciating the relationship between postnatal Qi, our external environment, our experiences, and emotions, will help you understand their role in the production of Blood and the circulation of experiences and emotions by the Heart.

It is through our blood that we are nourished. We can view our body as a vessel that shows where we have been. Since Blood is pumped through the Heart, it is imperative to the daily decisions we make in life that nourish our being or cause conflict.

The Yellow Emperor's Classic of Medicine (also know as the Huang di Nei Jing Su Wen), circa 240 BCE, is a foundational text of Chinese medicine. It is a dialog between the emperor and his acupuncturist, Qi Bo. It states that "the liver receives blood so there is sight; the legs receive blood, and thus are able to walk; the hands receive blood and are able to grip; the fingers receive blood and are able to grasp...."

Blood has a direct relationship to Qi. So if Qi is vacuous (see page 13) it will affect Blood; if Blood is stagnant there will likely be Qi stagnation.

It is through our blood that we are nourished.

Meridians and Acupressure Points

Meridians are pathways that transport Qi and Blood, regulate Yin and Yang, resist pathogens, reflect the signs and symptoms of a patient, transmit needling sensations, and regulate deficiency and excess conditions.

The classic Chinese medical text known as the Huang Emperor's Canon of Eighty-One Difficult Issues (Huangdi Bashiyi Nan Jing), circa 1st century CE, states that "the channels move Blood and Qi and ensure the free flow of Yin and Yang, so that the body is properly nourished." All parts of the body, through the meridians, form an integrated, unified whole.

Along these meridians are acupressure or acupuncture points (also known as energetic points). Acupressure points are "energy centers" that can be used as a means of engaging the body's natural healing capability. The body has a scientifically verified and measurable amount of electrical current flowing through it. The most active sites of electrical activity occur around the same areas that are deemed acupressure points. There are approximately 361 main acupressure points, although many more minor acupressure points also exist.

Acupressure points have precise functions, and these functions coincide with those of essential oils. When applying essential oils to these energy centers we guide ourselves to move toward a new, healthier way of being. The choice of which meridian and acupressure point to use will determine which direction of healing the body is to take. When teaching acupuncturists, I always explain that needles do not have an inherent personality or function; they are dependent upon the practitioner's Qi and the adaptability of the client. Therefore, in many cases it is better to simply use essential oils.

THE TWELVE MAJOR MERIDIANS

There are twelve major meridians on the body that circulate and balance our Qi. Each meridian pertains to a specific organ and element. The Yin meridians (Lung, Pericardium, Heart, Spleen, Liver, and Kidney) are located on the inner surfaces of the limbs and on the chest and abdomen. The Yang meridians (Large Intestine, San Jiao, Small Intestine, Urinary Bladder, Gall Bladder, and Stomach) are located on the outer surfaces of the limbs, and over the back, buttocks, and hips. The twelve major meridians are mirrored on both sides of the body.

All the major meridians can be accessed through the Qi found on the surface of the body. As the meridians move closer to the trunk from the extremities, they are said to move deeper and deeper inside the body, eventually hitting their organ. Therefore, each meridian's connection to its organ is direct.

All the meridians either start or end at the fingers or toes, and it is at these points that one meridian connects to another meridian. The fingers or toes are also where the meridian is considered most superficial. It is said that the Lungs distribute the Qi, which starts in the abdomen and goes through the Lung meridian. From there it travels to the Large Intestine, then to the Stomach, Spleen, Heart, Small Intestine, Urinary Bladder, Kidney, Pericardium, San Jiao, Gall Bladder, and finally completes its cycle through the body with the Liver. It then starts again with the Lungs. If one looks at where each meridian ends and where the subsequent meridian begins, one will find that they are in close proximity, making it easy for Qi to navigate the meridian changes.

Meridians are pathways that transport Qi and Blood.... Acupressure points are "energy centers" that can be used as a means of engaging the body's natural healing capability.

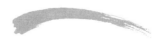

MAJOR MERIDIANS

Meridian	Abbreviation
Lung	LU
Spleen	SP
Small Intestine	SI
Kidney	KD
Liver	LV
Du	DU
Ren	RN

The first and last meridian points that are visible on these diagrams are labeled here. Some points cannot be seen on these views of the body.

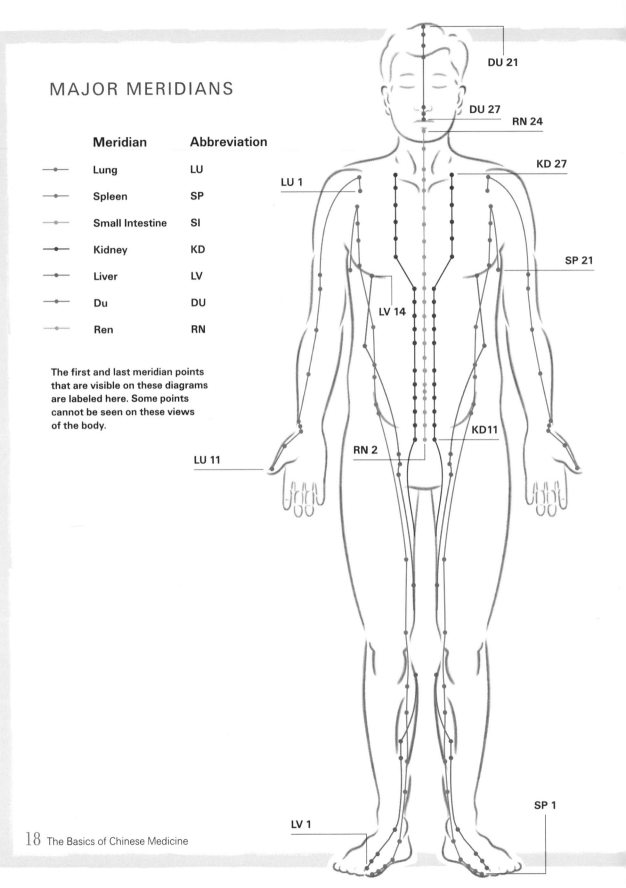

DU 21
DU 27
RN 24
KD 27
LU 1
SP 21
LV 14
KD11
SP 1
RN 2
LU 11
LV 1

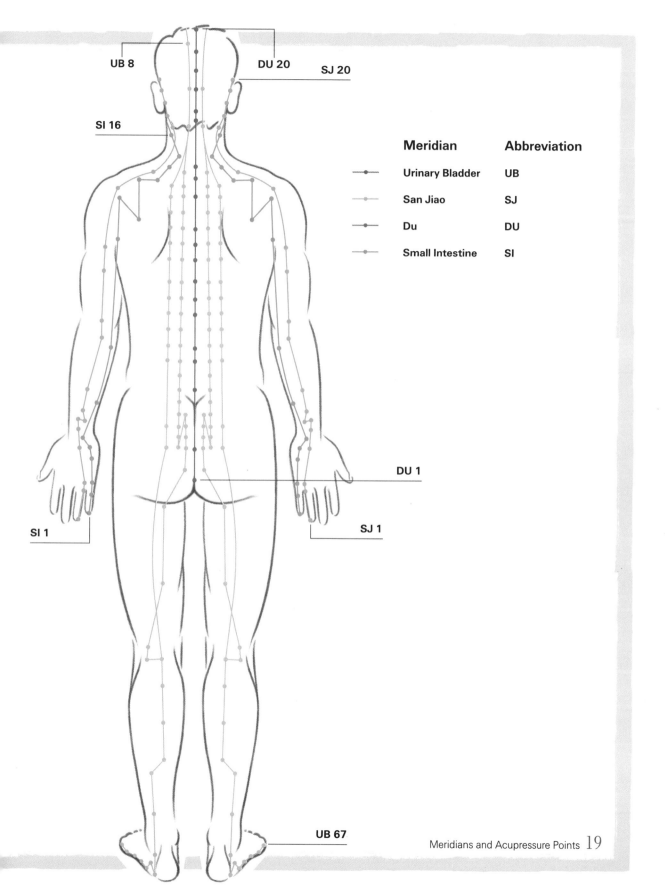

UB 8

DU 20

SJ 20

SI 16

Meridian	Abbreviation
Urinary Bladder	UB
San Jiao	SJ
Du	DU
Small Intestine	SI

DU 1

SI 1

SJ 1

UB 67

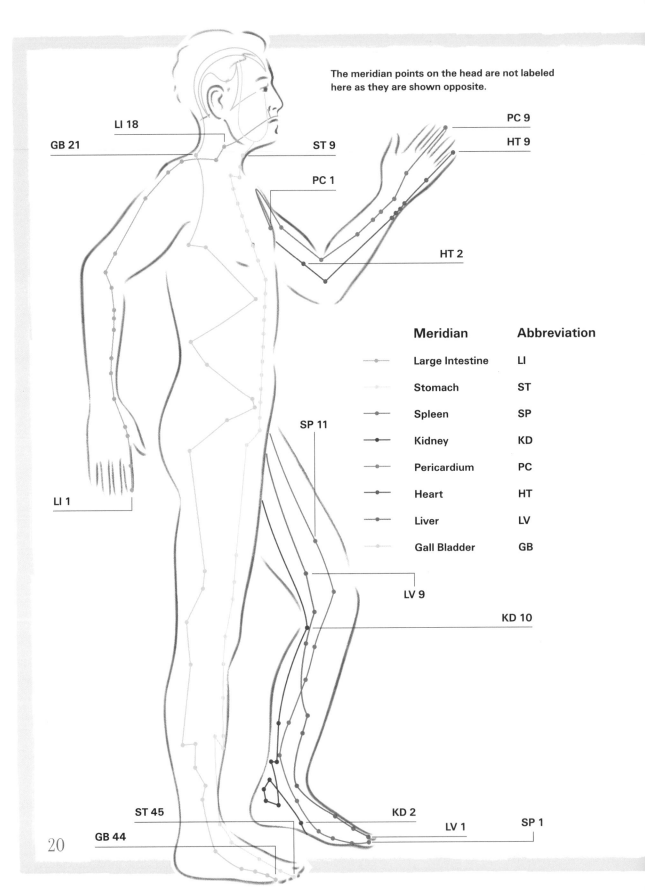

The meridian points on the head are not labeled here as they are shown opposite.

LI 18

GB 21

ST 9

PC 9

HT 9

PC 1

HT 2

SP 11

LI 1

LV 9

KD 10

Meridian	Abbreviation
Large Intestine	LI
Stomach	ST
Spleen	SP
Kidney	KD
Pericardium	PC
Heart	HT
Liver	LV
Gall Bladder	GB

ST 45

GB 44

KD 2

LV 1

SP 1

Meridian	Abbreviation	Meridian	Abbreviation
Large Intestine	LI	San Jiao	SJ
Stomach	ST	Gall Bladder	GB
Small Intestine	SI	Du	DU
Urinary Bladder	UB	Ren	RN

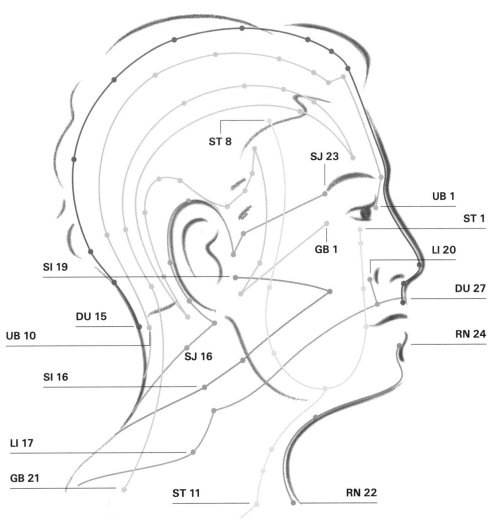

CUTANEOUS MERIDIANS

The cutaneous meridians have no acupressure points, they are simply twelve areas that lie superficially on the skin's surface, one representing each of the twelve major meridians. The cutaneous meridians serve to protect the internal environment from the exterior. They hold the Wei Qi (see page 14), and they are important when we Release the Exterior.

TENDINOMUSCULAR MERIDIANS

The tendinomuscular meridians (also known as the sinew meridians) circulate the Wei Qi and strengthen the articulation of joints. These meridians have no acupressure points, and they are broader than the primary meridians as they are the muscles, tendons, and ligaments associated with each of the twelve major meridians. The tendinomuscular meridians are mainly used to treat musculoskeletal conditions. When massage techniques are applied, we often use the tendinomuscular meridians.

EXTRAORDINARY MERIDIANS

There are eight extraordinary meridians that act as reservoirs of Qi. These channels can be tapped into at points on the major organ meridians, but they are not associated with the major meridians. According to Li Shi Zhen in the Study of the Eight Extraordinary Vessels, when there is excess Qi in the major meridians, the extraordinary meridians take up the excess in order to warm the organs internally and irrigate the space between the skin and muscles externally. For our purposes, the two extraordinary meridians we will be working with are the Ren and Du channels.

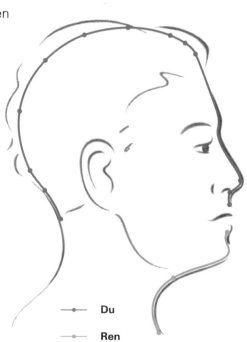

TWELVE DIVERGENT MERIDIANS

The twelve divergent meridians strengthen the connection between Yin and Yang organs and the major meridians. They integrate areas of the body not covered by the major meridians and also act as a second line of defense from evil Qi. They travel to the face.

—•— **Du**

—•— **Ren**

Jing

Jing (also known as essence) is the rich storehouse of energy that our bodies need in order to grow and develop from a fetus to an adult, to maintain normal organ function, and to reproduce. Everything our body does and experiences is dependent on Jing.

Our Jing is passed to us from our ancestors. At the moment of our conception, a part of our parents' Jing is combined through their sperm and egg. Once the egg is fertilized, development occurs rapidly, fueled by this initial spark of energy. We enter the world with this reserve of Jing, and our storehouse of Jing is nourished or depleted by our experiences, choices, trials, and traumas.

Our Jing resides deep within the physical body, and it travels through our organs and tissues via the major meridians and their many small branches. As we use Jing to support physical activity (conscious or unconscious), mental concentration, and emotional exchange it rises toward the surface tissues of the body and its nature becomes more active. This electrical energy response is called Qi. We can see Qi in the motility of the gut, the beating of the heart, and an electric surge or nerve response, and it also supports our consciousness, mental clarity, and emotional landscape. When our storehouse of Jing is full, it reaches all the areas of the body's tissues and fully supports all activities. However, growth and function will suffer when our Jing is weak.

There are three types of Jing: prenatal Jing, postnatal Jing, and Kidney Jing.

PRENATAL JING AND PRENATAL QI

Prenatal Jing is the nutritive source energy that we acquire from our parents. When the sperm and the egg join, it brings together the most potent fountainhead of energy from each parent, as well as from the entire ancestral lineage on both sides of the family. This initial spark of Prenatal Jing not only nourishes the embryo during pregnancy but also supplies us with the energy we need for all bodily functions and growth throughout life. In this way we all come into the world with a full savings account of energy resources to work with, and we are entrusted to live a balanced life that does not drain our store of Jing too heavily.

As soon as fertilization occurs, this newly joined matter starts to grow and divide. The first cleaving into two cells forms the Ren and Du meridians (see opposite). These are the deepest reservoirs of Yin and Yang in the body. As the fetus continues to develop, so does the rest of the meridian system. As the meridian system becomes more developed and extends into all areas and levels of the body, the prenatal Jing begins to flow into the system to fuel continuing expansion.

The prenatal Jing flowing throughout the meridians is called prenatal Qi. While there are several categories of Qi in the body with specific functions, Qi always refers to the active energy of the body. The Chinese character for Qi is made up of pictograms showing a bowl of rice with steam coming off of it. The solid food is the aspect of substance while the steam and the unseen nutrients of the food are the active aspect of the rice. Prenatal Jing is the nutritive substance we all harbor and utilize for all of our life functions, while prenatal Qi is the electric "steam" from this source that travels through the meridians.

Prenatal Qi is closely related to the health of our parents and ancestors. Therefore, inherited illnesses and behavior patterns are associated with this Qi. Prenatal Qi is also associated with our soul, determining our constitution and our life lessons.

Prenatal Qi energy cannot be replaced but it can be conserved with proper use of postnatal Qi (see below), depending on a healthy diet, environment, exercise, Qigong, work, and moderate sexual activity.

POSTNATAL JING AND POSTNATAL QI

While we are born with a store of prenatal Jing, we still have the responsibility to preserve and grow what we are given. Our lifestyle choices, including the foods we eat, our activities, and emotional stressors, all work to chip away at or to add to our store of Jing. Any Jing that we add to this store after birth is called postnatal Jing.

The postnatal Jing that flows through the meridians is called postnatal Qi (also known as acquired Qi). Returning to the pictograms for the Chinese character for Qi, the foundation for supporting healthful energy in the body is through good food. The foods we eat are processed efficiently and the useable nutrients are extracted. In this way we continuously work to create more postnatal Jing, which enables more postnatal Qi to flow into all parts of the body.

If our lifestyle practices are poor, or if we experience overwhelming stress, trauma, or habits like addiction, this will deplete our store of Jing. In this situation the body is not efficiently creating postnatal Jing, and more of our continuous energy needs are being pulled from our store of prenatal Jing. When this type of "overspending" occurs, it can result in areas of lowered function in the body, manifesting as retarded growth and development, premature aging, infertility, or problems with the bones, nervous system, or brain function.

Our postnatal Qi may also come from experiences in our external environment (relationships, work, or things we see in the media, for example) that move through the Wei level to the Ying level (see page 30). Most often, postnatal Qi is associated with habits and choices. Inhaling certain essential oils can quickly change thought patterns and help us make better lifestyle choices.

Jing is the rich storehouse of energy that our bodies need to grow and develop from a fetus to an adult, to maintain normal organ function, and to reproduce.

The Spleen and Stomach transform postnatal Qi into internal nourishment and Qi. This transformative process depends on not only the strength of the Spleen and Stomach but also the warming function of the Kidneys. In short, Kidney Qi supports all the functions of the body. Essential oils that support the transformation and transportation of postnatal Qi are those that warm and strengthen Spleen and Kidney Qi, such as sweet fennel, coriander, rosemary, cinnamon bark, clove, and ginger.

KIDNEY JING AND KIDNEY QI

The Kidney meridian system houses the body's Jing store (both prenatal and postnatal Jing). When our store of Jing is abundant, fertility and reproduction is possible. Essential oils that support the reproductive process have an affinity for the Kidney meridian system, and their viscous, nutritive nature supports the inclination of the body to gather and store Jing in order to maintain fertility and optimal function. This refers to both the preservation of prenatal Jing and the efficient processing of food (and other lifestyle factors) into postnatal Jing. While Jing remains abundant,

Rosemary

prenatal and postnatal Qi flow equally through the meridian system and support all of the body's functions.

This gathering of Jing by the Kidney meridian system is referred to as the Dan Tien, loosely translated as "Elixir Field." The Dan Tien is not confined to the physical kidney organ or the Kidney meridian system, but rather to the entire lower abdomen below the navel (see illustration below). This formless conglomeration of energy is what martial artists and those practicing Qigong and other energy practices call upon to perform amazing feats. Vibrational therapies such as aromatherapy, acupuncture, and healing touch modalities also access this storehouse of Jing for healing. Even without specialized training, all of us rely on the gathering of Jing in the Dan Tien for our bodies' constant daily functions, growth, and development.

Kidney Jing is a mixture of prenatal Jing and postnatal Jing that is stored in the Kidneys. It has a deep and viscous fluid nature. Kidney Jing is associated with the cycles of life and our paths unfolding, and it also produces marrow. Kidney Qi is formed when Kidney Jing combines with Kidney Yin and Kidney Yang. Symptoms of Kidney Jing deficiency include premature aging, infertility, impotence, feelings of internal cold, and apathy.

Jing and prenatal Qi are associated with thick and viscous essential oils like spikenard, vetiver, and myrrh. These oils often have a heavy and at times overwhelming scent. The reason that these oils can be overwhelming is that prenatal Qi and Jing are associated with our subconscious mind.

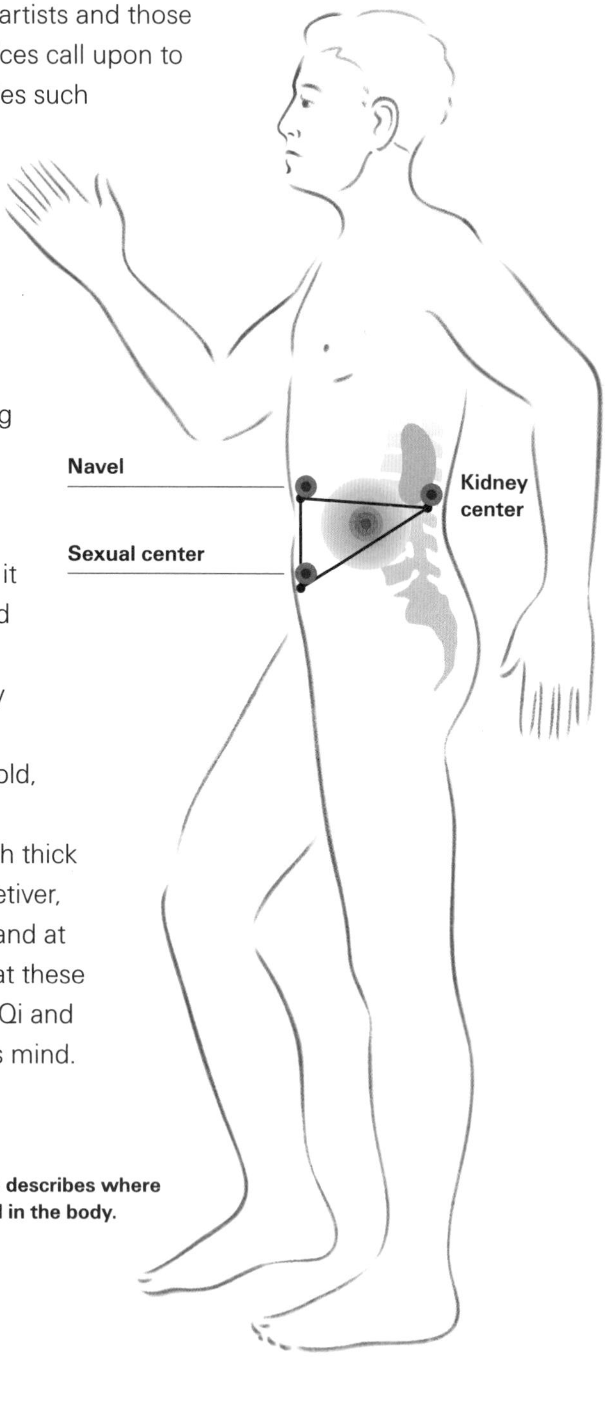

Navel

Sexual center

Kidney center

The Dan Tien describes where Jing is stored in the body.

Shen

It has been my experience that when clients take in the scent of different aromas their moods and thereby their decisions and actions can shift. Certain aromas, such as lavender and Roman chamomile, can induce relaxation and calm, while others, such as rosemary and basil, can evoke a sense of self-determination and confidence. In terms of Chinese medicine, aromatherapy has a direct relationship and effect on the Shen.

Basil

The Shen is equated to the mind and it resides in the Heart. Chinese Medicine believes that all disease is rooted in the mind-heart. Therefore, when using aromatherapy, we have the ability to work on the symptom and the root of illness. A plethora of self-help books affirm that by changing the mind we can change our environment. What if we complement that by the inhalation of certain aromas that have been proven to elevate our moods, emotions, and physical body? In order to understand this possibility, let's see how it relates to the Shen.

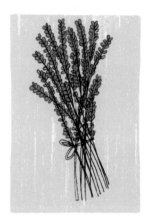

Lavender

The Shen is thought of as the spirit or consciousness. It resides in the Heart, which is known as the king or the sovereign ruler of the body. The Shen is also known as the motivating force behind our decisions and our personality. Why, when, and how we make decisions are all based on the Shen. In a religious context, it is believed that there are no accidents and all is in the right place at the right time. Yet in a medical context, it is thought that decisions are a cause of illness. What we choose to eat, where we choose to live, who we choose to associate ourselves with, who we will not forgive, and which past actions we will not forgive are all choices that we make, often in relation to what is driving and motivating us according to our personality.

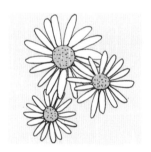

Roman chamomile

The Heart stores the Shen. The function of the Heart is to propel or circulate the Blood, which contains our emotions and experiences. Patients will often feel like they are looking for a way out, or a way to escape the past. The problem is that the Heart is circulating the same Blood and emotions from past experiences, and the Shen is making the same choices that are responsible for where the person is in his or her life, or the phase of evolution in which they are stuck.

The Shen in Chinese medicine is equated to the mind and resides in the Heart. Chinese Medicine believes that all disease is rooted in the mind-heart.

Just as a king is responsible for proper choices and actions for his land, so our mind or Shen is responsible for the choices we make in life. To be sovereign is to have authority over oneself regardless of outside influences, to have an awareness of what we are here to accomplish, and a sense to remain within our own integrity and authenticity. When the Shen or Heart is disturbed, the choices made are not the best for the body. So we can see that our choices have a direct relationship to our health.

When we inhale aromas we are awakening and opening the orifices of our being and beginning to awaken our spirit to new possibilities. From a TCM perspective, this will clear away Phlegm (see page 89) and Dampness (see page 39) that has been inhibiting our decision-making. Hence, we can move in a healthier and more positive direction.

We are all in the process of becoming, and it is my goal that the information in this book will inspire you to begin to take steps toward your own healing and to live a life with deeper purpose: a life where you feel connected to your soul.

Chapter 2

Classifying Essential Oils based on Chinese Medicine

According to Traditional Chinese Medicine (TCM), essential oils can be classified in four different ways. Exploring these classification systems will help you to understand how best to use individual oils.

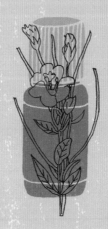

The Three Levels of Qi

The three levels of Qi (consciousness/experience) are Wei Qi, Ying Qi, and Yuan Qi. In aromatherapy terms, these levels relate to the fragrance notes of essential oils: the top notes, middle notes, and base notes respectively.

THE WEI LEVEL

The Wei level is associated with the outer and most superficial level of our consciousness and experience. Wei level oils have a close relationship with our lungs and breath. Like the wind, these essential oils are the most volatile and have an effect on acute conditions of the upper body. Oils with top notes include all the essential oils that are distilled from peels and many that are distilled from leaves. Common examples are lemon, orange, peppermint, and *Eucalyptus radiata*. Top notes are often used for treating common colds, to quickly uplift someone's mood by diffusing or inhaling the oil, or as a refresher at the end of a massage treatment. Wei level oils are the least thick, or viscous, of all the essential oils. They evaporate quickly, typically within 45 minutes to 2 hours. They do not penetrate the Ying or Yuan levels.

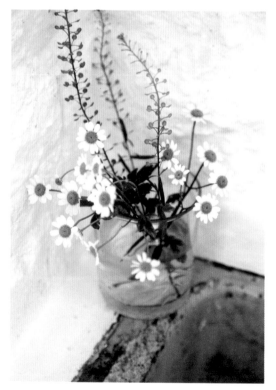

Chamomile

THE YING LEVEL

From the external Wei level we move to the Ying level. The Ying level is associated with organ Qi, postnatal Qi, Blood, and emotions. Essential oils that have the ability to strengthen our immune and digestive systems and support our muscular system are associated with the Ying level. These oils are middle notes, and they last longer than top notes. Ying level oils include tea tree, which is famous for its ability to tonify and strengthen the Lung Qi; Roman chamomile, which is highly regarded as one of the best oils to use to support the digestive system; and lemongrass (also known as the tendinomuscular oil), which helps to promote the movement of Qi and alleviate muscular pain.

THE YUAN LEVEL

The deepest and most mysterious level is that of Yuan Qi —the Yuan (source) level. This level is closely associated with DNA and our potential, and it is connected to our Jing. Oils with base notes are derived from resins, woods, and roots, as well as some flowers, and they are the thickest essential oils. They are often used to treat chronic conditions and are also great to use for descending our Qi (directing our energy downward). Yuan level oils are associated with the most Yin aspect of our being, they are often used to treat symptoms that manifest in the evening hours, such as insomnia and night sweats. I recommend applying these oils in the evening as this correlates with their Yin nature and will improve their effectiveness. Common examples are spikenard, sandalwood, vetiver, and rose.

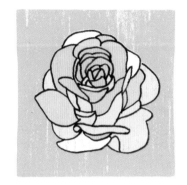

Rose

UNDERSTANDING THE THREE LEVELS

Level of Qi	Traditional aromatherapy classification	Association	Common usage
Wei Level	Top note oils	Outer consciousness and experience	Colds, mood uplifter, refresher
Ying Level	Middle note oils	Organ Qi, blood, and emotions	Immune system, digestive system, muscular system
Yuan-Source Level	Base note oils	DNA and potential	Insomnia, night sweats, reproductive system, grounding, meditation

The Five Elements

Another method of classifying essential oils is based on Five-Elements theory. The Five Elements are Wood, Fire, Earth, Metal, and Water. Five-Element theory was developed during the Han dynasty (206 BCE–220 CE), and it can be used to depict various universal events and interactions, including astrology, military agendas, seasons, times of day, and disease states. Five-Element theory is a great asset when you need to discover the overall constitution of an individual.

   We are all born with one or two dominant elements that dictate most of our responses to situations in life. In addition to our dominant elements, we also have aspects of the other elements as non-dominant characteristics. The Qi of each

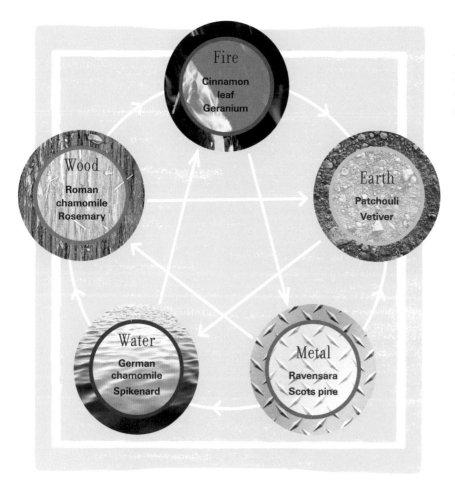

This shows how the Five Elements act upon each other and includes the associated essential oils.

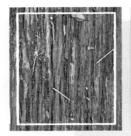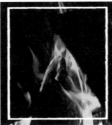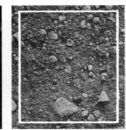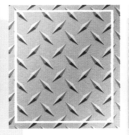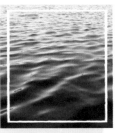

FIVE ELEMENT ASSOCIATIONS

	WOOD	FIRE	EARTH	METAL	WATER
Yin organ and meridian	Liver	Heart, Pericardium	Spleen	Lung	Kidney
Yang organ and meridian	Gall Bladder	Small Intestine, San Jiao	Stomachs	Large Intestine	Bladder
Season	Spring	Summer	Late summer	Fall (autumn)	Winter
Climate	Wind	Heat	Dampness	Dryness	Cold
Color	Green	Red	Yellow	White	Deep blue
Emotions	Anger, resentment	Excess joy, anxiety	Worry, pensiveness	Grief, integrity	Fear, courage
Sound	Shouting	Laughter	Singing	Weeping	Groaning
Body part	Tendons	Pulse	Muscle	Skin	Bones
Sense	Eyes	Tongue	Mouth	Nose	Ears
Taste	Sour	Bitter	Sweet	Pungent	Salty

element rises and falls depending on the season, time of day, and external factors such as our diet and relationships. Throughout our life we will need to either strengthen our non-dominant traits or soothe or engage our dominant ones.

The element that is most predominant in ourselves makes up what is called our constitution. This correlates to our Yuan Qi. We can think of our constitution as the lens through which we view the world, experience it, and make choices. "Healing" often begins with an understanding of the elements in our constitution and can eventually lead to living a life of awareness and acceptance of our being.

In Chinese medicine terms, an excess expression of our dominant traits is referred to as "excessive," while qualities that are not abundant are described as "deficient." In

PERSONALITY TRAITS AND PHYSICAL AILMENTS

ELEMENT	PERSONALITY TRAITS
Wood	Driven and determined, goal-oriented, controlling, a planner, desires to be challenged, prone to frustration and anger. **If excessive**: always needs to be in control, inflexible, doesn't work well with others in groups (unless the leader), becomes frustrated when things do not move quickly enough. **If deficient**: unable to make plans, poor judgment, timidity, low self-confidence.
Fire	Inspirational, charismatic, creative, joyful, easily excited, finds it easy to have ideas but difficult to put them into practice, sensitive, a dreamer, passionate, can be a social butterfly. **If excessive**: impulsive, explosive anger, excessive talking, easily stimulated. **If deficient**: daydreaming, lack of self-expression, low self-confidence and drive, feels as if he or she has nothing to give to others or share with the world, easily frightened.
Earth	Intelligent and focused when working, reliable, nurturing, mothering, wants everyone and everything to be okay, takes on other people's problems. **If excessive**: obsessive compulsive, overbearing to others. **If deficient**: prone to worry, needy, clingy, desires to feel accepted, over-nurturing, not grounded, pensive, desire for sympathy.
Metal	Organized, intellectual, disciplined, efficient. **If excessive**: authoritative, insensitive, seeks perfection, very orderly, selfish, exceptionally clean and organized, defensive, critical. **If deficient**: melancholy, disorganized, careless, trouble letting go, dislike of speaking.
Water	Strong, courageous, introspective, an observer, cautious, mindful, philosophical, deep. **If excessive**: impatient, focused on their legacy. **If deficient**: weak, fearful, low motivation.

the Personality Traits and Physical Ailments chart below, essential oils that are labeled "deficiency" can be used to bring out qualities that are lacking or dormant, while oils that are labeled "excess" can be used to transform a trait to another element.

One of the virtues of using Five-Element theory to look at life is that it helps us to cool our judgment and allows us to observe both ourselves and other people with compassion and acceptance. If we understand that everyone is born with a specific constitution that needs to move through experiences in order to complete the soul in this particular life cycle, then we can live knowing that we are all in the process of becoming.

COMMON PHYSICAL AILMENTS	ESSENTIAL OILS
If excessive: bloating, rib-side pain, muscular tightness, migraines. **If deficient**: hernias, brittle nails, tight sinews, blurry vision, mood swings.	**For excess**: *Lavandula angustifolia*, Roman chamomile. **For deficiency**: rosemary, lemongrass.
If excessive: sweating, a red face, feeling ungrounded, easily stimulated, restless. **If deficient**: easily frightened, feeling ungrounded, lack of desire for new experiences, speech difficulties such as stuttering, poor circulation, shortness of breath, sweating.	**For excess**: geranium, German chamomile, lavender. **For deficiency**: cinnamon leaf, melissa, neroli, rosemary.
If excessive: feeling of fullness and heavyness, easily gains weight. **If deficient**: sweet cravings, lethargy, loose stools or constipation, weight gain, weight loss.	**For excess and deficiency**: rosemary, patchouli, coriander, neroli.
If excessive: nasal and chest congestion, loud cough with phlegm, constipation, feeling of distention in lower abdomen, constriction of chest muscles. **If deficient**: frequent colds, spontaneous sweating, asthma, nasal congestion, shortness of breath, pale complexion, easily fatigued, constipation.	**For excess**: *Lavandula angustifolia*, *Eucalyptus radiata*, *Eucalyptus globulus*. **For deficiency**: ravensara, tea tree, Scots pine.
If excessive: not applicable. **If deficient**: frequent urination, urgent bowel movements, lower body edema, cold and achy lower back, knee and ankle pain, history of bone fractures, ringing in ears, low libido, asthma, arthritis.	**For excess**: not applicable. **For deficiency**: ginger, Scots pine, cypress, cinnamon bark, cedarwood.

TCM Function

Practitioners of Chinese herbal medicine and acupuncture rely on specific TCM functions to guide them in choosing herbs and acupuncture points. The functions of essential oils can be classified in a similar way—by taste, temperature, meridian or body system affinity, and what parts of the plant are used (see page 40).

While this book does not support the internal use of essential oils, it is important to understand that essential oils used for aromatherapy purposes are simply concentrated distillations of medicinal herbs, and there is much overlap between the plants used to make medicinal teas and those distilled for essential oils.

CLEARING HEAT

Clearing Heat is the treatment strategy to use in circumstances where there are symptoms of heat and inflammation, for example when a recent injury is red and inflamed. It can also be used to treat insomnia, anger, red eyes, and a red face. Heat is associated with Yang, and it has a rising nature, like Fire. Examples of essential oils that clear and cool Heat are lavender, Roman chamomile, and ylang-ylang.

PROMOTING THE MOVEMENT OF QI

Promoting the movement of Qi is the treatment strategy to use when there is Qi stagnation (see page 12). Symptoms of Qi stagnation depend on the organ or meridian involved. Examples of Qi stagnation include physical pain of a dull nature, constipation, tight muscles, frequent sighing, emotional depression, and the feeling of being stuck in life. In short, promoting the movement of Qi aims to unblock the Qi, which will allow the person to feel more free. Examples of essential oils that promote the movement of Qi include lavender, lemongrass, rosemary, and peppermint.

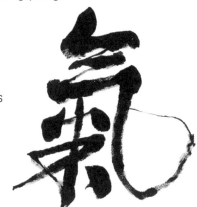

The External Factors of Illness

In Chinese medicine there are six external factors of illness, also known as the external pathogenic influences. Wind, Heat, Fire, and Dryness are all Yang pathogens while Cold and Dampness are Yin pathogens. Exterior conditions are those that affect the Wei level—the most external Qi of the body (see page 30), but if the pathogens are left unresolved then they will penetrate into the Interior and cause more harm.

Wind: Known as the chief of the one hundred diseases, Wind is wandering and changeable. It is said to bring the other pathogens inside, hence the combinations of Wind-Cold and Wind-Heat.

Cold: Cold is mostly experienced in the winter, and it often arises when people work or live in a cold environment. Cold causes constriction, just imagine how we naturally tighten our muscles when we go outside in the cold. Cold will also close pores (which is why in Wind-Cold there is not sweating). Cold can also lead to pain in the muscles and the joints.

Heat: This pathogen is seen in the summer or in hot climates. Major symptoms of Heat include profuse sweating, high fever, a red face, a decrease in bodily fluids, constipation, and dark yellow urine. Heat disorders often combine with Dampness.

Dryness: Dryness is usually experienced in the fall (autumn) and winter, and in dry climates. Its most common symptoms are dry hair, dry eyes, dry lips, dry throat, dry stools, thirst, and reduced urination.

Fire: Fire often affects the upper body, as heat rises and is considered Yang. Common symptoms include a red face, red skin, rashes, excess sweating (heat dries the sweat, leading to dryness), restlessness, and agitation.

Dampness: Dampness is heavy and tends to sink downward, causing heaviness of the limbs, sluggish digestion, water retention, bloating, a distended abdomen, heavy-headedness, and muddled thinking. Dampness tends to linger and is hard to resolve. In Western medicine, Dampness is often known as arthritis. Dampness can be divided into Damp-Cold and Damp-Heat.

TONIFYING THE QI

Tonifying the Qi is the treatment strategy to use when there are symptoms of Qi deficiency (see page 12). The word "tonify" means to strengthen and build. Symptoms of Qi deficiency depend on the organ involved. Major symptoms include lethargy, weakness of the limbs, feeling cold, loose stools, spontaneous sweating, low libido, lower back pain, frequent urination, and a pale face. Examples of essential oils that tonify the Qi include ravensara, tea tree, neroli, rosemary, and Scots pine.

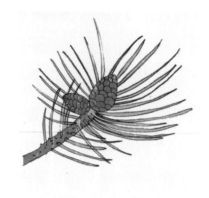

Scots pine

TONIFYING THE YANG

Yang energy supplies the body with the ability to perform its actions. Qualities of Yang energy include warmth, strength, fortitude, and transformation. Symptoms of Yang deficiency include lower back pain, frequent urination, edema in the lower extremities, weight gain, feeling cold, weak and flaccid muscles, low libido, lack of willpower, lack of motivation, and muscle weakness. Examples of essential oils that tonify the Yang are ginger, rosemary, and cinnamon bark.

NOURISHING YIN

Yin is synonymous with nourishment. When there is sufficient Yin it counterbalances the rising nature of Yang. In other words, Yin anchors the Yang. When the Yin is deficient the Yang is not anchored. Symptoms of Yin deficiency may include mood swings, insomnia, nervousness, night sweats, hot flashes (flushes), dry eyes, dry skin, and dry nails. Examples of essential oils that nourish the Yin include geranium, ylang-ylang, vetiver, and rose.

Geranium

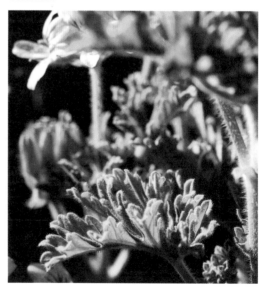

NOURISHING THE BLOOD

Blood is a fluid that nourishes the body. Blood is considered to be Yin, and the symptoms of Blood deficiency are similar to those of Yin deficiency. Common symptoms include dry skin, a pale and withered face, thinning hair, mood swings, insomnia, cold hands and feet, excess daydreaming, blurry vision, and dry eyes. Examples of essential oils that nourish the Blood are Roman chamomile and carrot seed.

INVIGORATING THE BLOOD

Invigorating the Blood is the treatment strategy to use when there are symptoms of Blood stagnation. In brief, Blood stagnation means that the blood is not flowing properly. Localized strains and sprains are common examples of Blood stagnation. Varicose veins, stabbing pains, and longstanding emotional stagnation are also forms of Blood stagnation. Examples of essential oils that invigorate the Blood include frankincense and melissa.

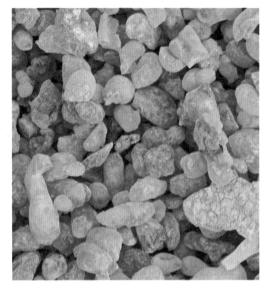

Frankincense resin

CALMING THE SHEN

This treatment strategy is used to treat a wide array of symptoms that involve our emotional nature. It attempts to bring calmness and reason to the mind. As the Shen is related to our mind and Heart, essential oils can be used to treat sleep issues, impulsivity, agitation, recklessness, and lack of mental order. Examples of essential oils that calm the Shen include lavender, geranium, and vetiver.

AROMATICALLY TRANSFORMING DAMPNESS

Transforming Dampness is the term used in Chinese medicine for alleviating the symptoms of Dampness. Dampness is a form of Qi stagnation that is the result of Spleen Qi deficiency. Eating cold and raw, hot and greasy foods, or very heavy foods is a major factor in developing Spleen Qi deficiency. Dampness can be divided into Damp-Cold and Damp-Heat. Whether it is a Damp-Cold or a Damp-Heat, major symptoms include heavinesss of limbs, sluggish digestion, water retention, bloating, a distended abdomen, heavy-headedness, and muddled thinking. Dampness can occur in all areas of the body. Most essential oils have the ability to treat Damp conditions. Examples of essential oils that aromatically transform Dampness include peppermint, rosemary, cardamom, lemon, and lemongrass.

The Parts of the Plant

The final way that essential oils can be classified is based on the parts of the plant that are used to make the oil. Novices often find this approach the easiest to grasp when starting out.

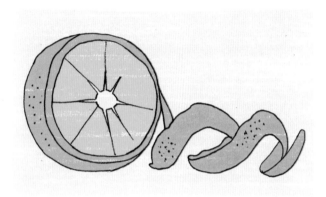

Orange

PEELS

Essential oils made from citrus peel, such as lemon, bergamot, grapefruit, and orange, are refreshing and inviting but their scents and effects are short-lived. These oils are top notes and they are wonderful to use in diffusers to help uplift the mood.

It is important to use a scent that is familiar and comforting the first time you use oils, or when making a blend for someone who is new to holistic healing, so oils derived from peels are an ideal choice as most people are familiar with citrus fragrances.

Oils derived from peels are excellent choices to use for symptoms of despondency because they can make you feel uplifted. However, these oils are top notes so they will not work on the deeper level of disease.

Essential oils from peels are cooling in nature so they can be used for acute Fire-Heat emotional symptoms, such as expressions of anger, anxiety, and lack of focus.

LEAVES

The majority of essential oils are derived from leaves. Compared to oils derived from peels, these oils have a bit more depth in their nature and functionality. Many leaves are prized for their antibacterial and antiviral properties. In fact, *Eucalyptus globulus* was often used during World War One to control outbreaks of meningitis.

Just as leaves are part of the upper and outer aspects of trees, so in Chinese medicine they are associated with the upper and outer aspects of our bodies: the head, neck, chest, arms, and lungs. Leaves take in carbon dioxide and let out oxygen, so it follows that oils derived from leaves are integral for conditions of the Lung.

The Lungs provide a direct link with our external environment and our Wei Qi (see page 14). After all, we take in breath through our nose—our most external orifice.

Oils derived from leaves are more effective and have longer-lasting effects than those derived from peels. They have the ability to tonify the Lung and Wei Qi, Release the Exterior, and address symptoms of the common cold, sinusitis, and rhinitis. However, they are most efficient in treating chest congestion and upper body aches. Oils with top notes, such as peppermint and *Eucalyptus radiata*, have the ability to open up the nasal passages, expel chest congestion, and are likely to be beneficial to bring relief to neck pain. Tea tree and ravensara, which are middle notes, have the ability to tonify the Lung Qi and Stabilize the Exterior (make strong, impenetrable boundaries that are not vulnerable to external pathogenic influence), making them beneficial to those people who frequently have common colds or spontaneous sweating.

Proficiency and order are the major characteristics of someone with strong Lung Qi. Such people are likely to have an upright posture—symbolizing the taking in of an abundant amount of life force. In contrast, people with chronic lung issues may be hunched over and not taking in enough oxygen. In other words, they are not taking in life force to be used in the present moment. This makes sense when we consider that the lungs are associated with grief: if the mind is living in the past, why does the body need an adequate amount of

Essential Oils and Mood Disorders

According to an article written in 2013 by researchers at Xiamen University, China: "Most studies, as well as clinically applied experience, have indicated that various essential oils, such as lavender, lemon, and bergamot can help to relieve stress, anxiety, depression, and other mood disorders. Most notably, inhalation of essential oils can communicate signals to the olfactory system and stimulate the brain to exert neurotransmitters (e.g. serotonin and dopamine) thereby further regulating mood."

Lavender

Tea tree

oxygen in the present? Oils that tonify the Lung Qi (and the Heart Qi), such as tea tree, ravensara, and eucalyptus, are also integral for those who tend toward sadness, grief, and nostalgia.

NEEDLES

Needles are similar to leaves. However, one important difference is that many oils derived from needles work with the Kidneys as well as the Lungs.

In Chinese medicine, full respiration relies on the relationship between Lung Qi and the Kidney Qi. As the Lungs inhale, the Qi from the oxygen is "grasped" by the Kidneys, which holds the Qi within the body. If the Kidney Qi or Jing is deficient this grasping quality will also be weak. Oils derived from needles, such as cypress and Scots pine, are excellent for assisting the Kidneys' ability to "grasp." Pine in particular can tonify the overall function of Kidney Qi.

It is also possible that the Kidneys may not "grasp" the Qi because the Lungs aren't supplying enough oxygen for the Kidneys to "grasp" properly. In such cases, oils derived from needles may help in tonifying the Lungs as well. Such oils are frequently used with frankincense to increase the depth of respiration.

Scots pine

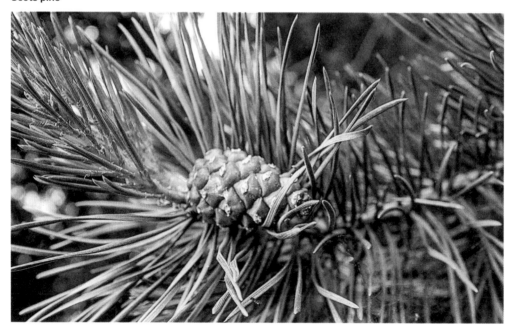

FLOWERS

Oils derived from flowers are some of the most expensive essential oils, and many people consider them to be the most sacred of oils. One of the reasons why floral oils cost so much is because flowers yield less oil than other parts of a plant. Another reason is the great amount of care and labor that must be used when distilling floral oils. Flowers often need to be picked during the early hours of the morning or at specific times of the year. When using floral oils, less is often more.

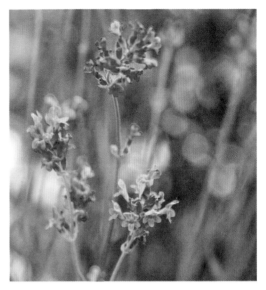

Floral oils are some of the most complex and nourishing of essential oils. Being feminine in nature, they are calming, cooling, and nourishing to the Yin. Inhaling these oils will easily soften the mood.

While oils derived from peels, leaves, and needles are associated with Releasing the Exterior, closing pores, and tonifying the Lung Qi, floral oils are associated with nourishing the Heart, Liver, and Kidneys.

Flowers such as lavender are often used for general relaxation and calmness. However, floral oils can be used for more than relaxation. For example, lavender can actually help to alleviate Plum Pit Qi (a sense that something is lodged in the throat, which is usually due to something that needs to be expressed); neroli is beneficial for loose stools

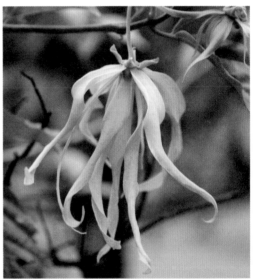

Top: Lavender
Bottom: Ylang-ylang

associated with anxiety; and ylang-ylang can be used for night sweats and hot flashes (flushes).

Just as flowers bloom in the spring and are a major component in pollination, so floral oils are practical to use for problems with the reproductive system and issues surrounding expressing creativity and sexuality.

RESINS

Oils derived from resins are associated with emotional and physical wounds that have not healed. We can understand this function from the way that resins are obtained: the trunk of a tree is slashed and the tree exudes a resin in an attempt to heal the wound. Resins are often used in creams and lotions for healing scar tissue, and they are also used with flowers for facial rejuvenation—antiaging. Oils derived from resins, especially frankincense, work very well with oils derived from needles to help the Kidneys "grasp" the Lung Qi.

ROOTS

Oils derived from roots are often the thickest and most viscous of essential oils, and they have the most mysterious aromas. They are extremely grounded and descending to our energy. As you can imagine, they are beneficial to be used on the lower aspects of the body, such as the soles of the foot, heels, and the base of the spine. These oils all have base notes, making them wise choices for chronic symptoms of insomnia, nervousness, anxiety, and fear. They are associated with Jing and the Kidneys, and will be a benefit to nourishing the Yin and calming the Shen. They may also be good for people who want to increase their attention span and cultivate more patience.

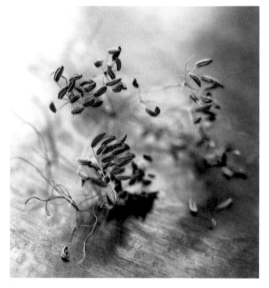

Fennel seeds

SEEDS

Oils derived from seeds have middle notes and are closely associated with the Spleen, Stomach, Liver, and Gall Bladder. Many of these oils benefit the transportation and transformation processes of the Spleen and Stomach and will aid in alleviating Dampness in these areas. They have the ability to tonify the Spleen, aromatically transform Dampness, and even nourish the Blood. Many of the seeds that are used in aromatherapy, such as coriander, fennel, and cardamom, can also be found in our kitchen cabinets. Metaphorically, seeds represent new starts and personal potential.

WOOD

Oils derived from wood have base notes, with the exception of rosewood, which is considered a middle note. These oils are associated with maturity of the mind and are beneficial for meditation and contemplation. This can be understood when one considers how long old trees can live and endure. Oils derived from wood are also associated with grounding, stability, and willpower. Common examples are sandalwood, cedarwood, and rosewood.

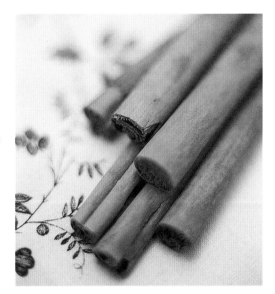

Cinnamon bark

BARK

Bark, the outer covering of a tree, is there to provide protection. It can be seen as a wall that inhibits anything from accessing the interior. Cinnamon bark, which is high in antiviral properties, can be used to stop pain. The warming nature of cinnamon bark makes it an ideal oil for joint pain that grows worse with cold.

The Doctrine of Signatures

In order to grasp the functions of an essential oil it is imperative to notice the physical characteristics, texture, shape, specific part distilled, and scent of the plant from which the oil is derived. This is known as the doctrine of signatures.

The concept dates back to Ancient Greece and the Greek botanist Dioscorides (40–90 CE) but its rise in popularity began in the Middle Ages. Paracelsus (1493–1541), a Swiss physician, philosopher, astrologer, and botanist, is quoted as saying "Nature marks each growth...according to its curative benefit." However, it was the German mystic Jakob Boehme (1575–1624) who is credited with further popularizing this concept in his book *Signatura Rerum* (The Signature of All Things), which was published in 1621. William Coles (1626–1662), a British botanist who heavily relied on the doctrine of signatures, took into consideration the whole plant or tree and the environment in which it grew.

PART 2

SELF-HEALING PRACTICES WITH AROMATHERAPY

Chapter 3

Using Essential Oils

In this chapter, we talk about the various ways that essential oils can be applied, and then learn more about the qualities of 28 essential oils.

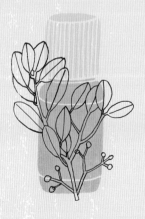

How to Use Essential Oils

Aromatherapy relies on the inhalation of essential oils, the external application of the oils, and the relationship between intention and willpower in order for people to make the positive changes necessary for healing. There are circumstances where essential oils are used internally, but this is done only under careful supervision.

INHALATION

Inhalation is the simplest way to use essential oils in their purest form. This method is the most effective way to absorb essential oils into the bloodstream, and it has the quickest effect on the limbic system, the structures in the brain that deal with emotions. The inhalation of aromas can induce calmness and relaxation and improve mental clarity and memory. For example, studies have shown that rosemary oil contains a compound called 1,8 cineole (see page 84) that can improve memory. It is interesting to note that this fact must have been known in William Shakespeare's time, as he writes in *Hamlet* (Act 4, Scene 5), "there's rosemary, that's for remembrance."

Inhaling oils is most beneficial for respiratory and emotional issues such as anxiety, insomnia, and palpitations. Certain oils can be inhaled for a mental tonic (peppermint and *Eucalyptus radiata*, for example), while others (such as geranium and palmarosa) will assist in inducing a state of peace—an almost grace-like state that lifts the spirit from day-to-day stressors and anxieties.

Methods of inhalation include placing a drop of oil on a cotton ball or a scarf or using an essential oil inhaler. Diffusing oils is another efficient method, but the effects are usually not as strong as direct inhalation. There are lots of different types of diffuser on the market, including candle, mist, and electric diffusers. Many of the mist diffusers can turn certain colors, so they are a good choice if you would like to add color therapy to your treatments.

Above: *Eucalyptus radiata*
Left: Palmarosa

Palm Inhalation Technique

This inhalation technique promotes relaxation and instigates the healing process. Gently massaging the palms of your hands activates the Pericardium 8 and Heart 8 acupressure points, both of which help to calm the mind and open our Heart energy, allowing us to become receptive to relaxation.

1 Put one drop of your chosen oil blend (see page 51) in the palm of your hand. Using your thumb or index finger, gently rub the oil into your palm for a few seconds..

2 Hold your hand, palm facing upward, about 4 inches (10 cm) away from your face. Slowly inhale through your nose to the count of six and then exhale completely through your mouth. Repeat three times. Yin and Yang are interdependent upon one another (you cannot have one without the other).

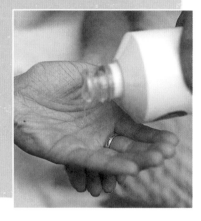

For insomnia, I recommend placing a drop of oil (palmarosa, geranium, lavender, Roman chamomile, and spikenard are all good choices) on your pillow on the top edge farthest away from your head (or on the pillow next to you if you have two pillows). Most often, all that is necessary to treat insomnia is to have a slight awareness of the scent. Why is this? Often the root of insomnia is subconscious, and at times strong scents can agitate the nervous system, even if they are intended to relax it. If you are looking to remember your dreams, try using rosemary oil.

If you are a massage therapist, chiropractor, or acupuncturist and are doing prone treatments, try putting a drop of bergamot, blood orange, lavender, peppermint, or *Eucalyptus radiata* oil on a cotton ball and then placing it on a chair under the face rest. If you use bergamot, blood orange, or lavender, your client is likely to have a very relaxing session, and may even fall asleep. On the other hand, using peppermint or *Eucalyptus radiata* will help to prevent your client's sinuses from becoming clogged. Another fun and simple option is to place a drop of an "awakening" oil, such as peppermint or *Eucalyptus radiata*, on a cotton ball and have the client inhale the aroma before they get up from the treatment table. This will help your client adjust to normal waking activity.

BATHS

I like to recommend baths to clients, particularly those who are new to holistic healing or have built up the physical and mental toxicity that can lead to a defensive character. This is because a bath can help one's spirit to become receptive, which is essential for getting the most from a healing journey. Baths symbolize a return to the womb, a place where we were completely receptive and in need of nutrients from our mother. Water is Yin (see page 10)—the nourishing and receptive aspect of our being.

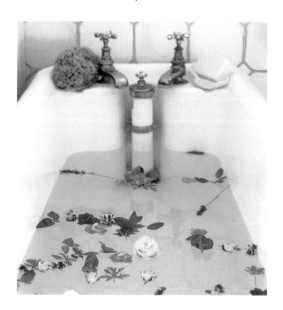

CAUTION: When bathing

Do not bathe with essential oils that are considered to be chemically hot, such as cinnamon and black pepper, as they will cause irritation. Also avoid oils with phenol constituents, including oregano, clove, and tansy.

Baths are very relaxing and can help people to achieve restful sleep. As the mind relaxes, so does the body, making a bath a great choice to help relieve muscle aches and pains. Baths can also help to eliminate toxins and alleviate the symptoms of the common cold and flu.

A simple way to add oils to your bath is to mix together 1 to 3 tablespoons liquid Castile soap with 4 to 6 drops of your chosen essential oil or blend of oils and then stir the mixture into a bathtub full of hot water. If you don't have liquid Castile soap then you can use salt. I like to add essential oils to ½ cup of Epsom salt or Himalayan sea salt and pour it into the water as the bath is filled. Another option is to substitute vegetable or jojoba oil (in the same quantity as liquid Castile soap), but to prevent it from floating on the surface of the water, agitate the water first to avoid any direct contact with the genitals.

The essential oils commonly used in baths are lavender, geranium, palmarosa, ravensara, tea tree, frankincense, sandalwood, vetiver, and patchouli.

Essential Oil Dilution Chart

You will need to dilute essential oils before you can apply them to your skin. This chart shows you how to prepare various dilutions of oils in bulk. For example, if you want to make a 5 percent dilution of a single essential oil in 2 teaspoons (10 ml) base oil, you need to add 15 drops of essential oil to the base oil.

To dilute a blend of essential oils, you need to divide the total number of drops of essential oil between however many essential oils you want to include in your blend. For example, if you want to make a 5 percent dilution of a blend of three essential oils in 2 teaspoons (10 ml) base oil, you would need to add 5 drops of each essential oil (15 drops in total) to the base oil.

Please note that using drops to blend oils is not an exact science and these quantities are approximate.

DILUTION PERCENTAGE	NUMBER OF DROPS			
5%	15	22	30	45
4%	12	18	24	36
3%	9	13	18	27
2%	6	9	12	18
1%	3	4	6	9
-5%	1	2	3	4
VOLUME OF BASE OIL	10ml	15ml ½ oz	20ml	30ml 1 oz

Chart based on an idea from the Tisserand Institute (tisserandinstitute.org) and used with permission.

DERMAL APPLICATION

Applying oils to the skin is another way to use essential oils. However, essential oils should be diluted with a base oil or cream before they are applied to the skin. Common base oils include jojoba, fractionated coconut (which can be a substitute for jojoba oil), sesame seed, arnica (see also page 129), and calendula oil.

Dermal application is very useful for pain relief. As you will discover, some oils are more beneficial than others for certain areas of the body. For example, peppermint is exceptional for neck pain, Scots pine and lemongrass are good for back and hip pain, and ginger is ideal for knee and ankle pain. I often like to apply a warm moist compress (see page 52) to the affected area before using a blend of oils to treat the pain.

My favorite way to use essential oils on the body is to apply them to acupressure points (see page 16). Acupressure points have precise functions and personalities

HOW TO MAKE AND USE A WARM MOIST COMPRESS

Compresses can be used to reduce inflammation and alleviate pain. They can be applied to areas that are too painful to massage, or used to relax the muscles before a massage. Most people find the effects of a warm compress to be relaxing and soothing. The benefit of using a moist compress, rather than a dry one, is that it increases the skin's permeability to essential oils.

You will need

Hand towel or washcloth (face flannel)
Towel

1 Soak a hand towel or washcloth (face flannel) in hot water—the water should only be as warm as you can comfortably stand. Wring out any excess water.
2 Place the compress over the affected area, cover with a dry towel, and leave it in place until the compress cools.

Tips for Using Essential Oils

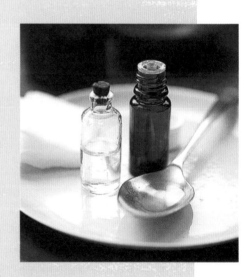

- Always store essential oils in a cool, dark place and keep them out of reach of children.
- Make sure bottle caps are sealed tightly.
- Store oils in amber or dark-colored bottles to protect them from light.
- Keep citrus and Scots pine oils in the refrigerator to preserve their freshness.
- Always use high-quality essential oils.
- Warm your body before applying oil. This will help your skin to absorb the oil. Try applying oil during or after showering or placing a warm moist compress on the skin after application.
- Make sure your skin is clean before applying oil—dirty skin will decrease the absorption rate.
- Do not let oils come into any contact with your eyes, genitals, or ear canals.

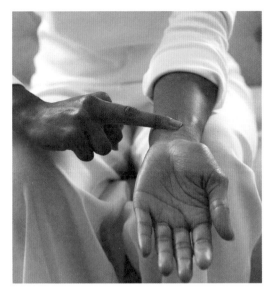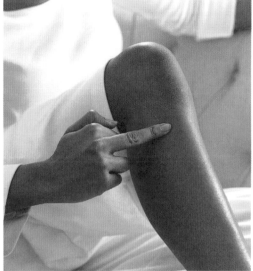

that directly correlate to the spirit and functions of essential oils. For example, lavender (*Lavandula angustifolia*) and the Pericardium 6 point both have the function to open up the chest and calm the Shen (see page 27); spikenard and the Kidney 1 point both have the function to descend the Qi; and lemongrass and the Gall Bladder 34 point are both influential to the muscles.

Please note: In the blends featured in chapters 4–7, the instructional artworks often show acupressure points on one side of the body. However, because the twelve major meridians are mirrored on both sides of the body (see page 17), you have the option to apply oil to these points on both sides of the body and I would recommend this for the most effective treatment.

Roll-on bottles

Although a dropper bottle is a very common way to store and apply essential oils, another option is a roll-on bottle. Roll-on bottles provide an easy way to apply essential oils and many people prefer them to dropper bottles.

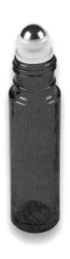

If you are applying essential oil on acupressure points using a roll-on bottle, you can gently press the tip of the bottle on the point and massage in the oil in a circular motion. Approximately five circles is 1 drop of oil, or if you are using it on meridians, you can simply apply up and/or down the meridian.

The roll-on bottle has many advantages, such as being easier to apply and more portable, and leaving less oil on your hand or finger and more oil on the desired area. However, please note that it is not as exact as a dropper bottle.

The Breath and Healing

The breath is associated with survival, healing, and the evolution of consciousness. It is both the beginning and the end of life. We come into this world with our first inhalation and we leave it with our final exhalation. We can live without food or water for an extended period of time but we cannot live without oxygen. Oxygen maintains life.

Those of us who have engaged in any kind of yoga, Qigong, breathwork, or meditation will have experienced how changing the speed and depth of our breathing can help us become mentally, emotionally, and physically more present, making us closer to our true nature.

It is my hope that your use of essential oils will be accompanied by a deepening of your own breathing patterns. For when you initiate healing with your breath, you are choosing to first change your consciousness with your own being and move closer to being your own healer.

Most people do not pay enough attention to how breathing influences their patterns of thought, emotions, and even behavior. The lungs and the heart have a direct relationship, meaning the depth of inhalation influences the rate of your heart. Therefore, as much as we look to outside means to calm the mind, cool anxiety, and reduce stress, alternating our breathing patterns may create the best "cure."

Shallow breathing, stressful experiences, and negative thoughts keep our sympathetic nervous system in high gear. This can lead to an overuse of our adrenals, which can be accompanied by symptoms of anxiety, insomnia, mood

BE MORE PRESENT

This breathing exercise should help you to feel calm, relaxed, and more present. It can also help to improve your mental clarity and focus and stimulate creativity. Try it out and see for yourself if you notice a change.

1 Sit in a comfortable position, preferably with your spine aligned and straight.

2 Start by taking slow, deep breaths to the count of six, exhaling completely through your mouth. Do this three times.

3 Continue to take slow, deep breaths. As you do so, slowly state in your mind, "Calmness within my mind. Balance within my body. Unity in my mind, body, and spirit." Repeat this mantra at least three times.

"For breath is life, and if you breathe well you will live long on earth."

Sanskrit proverb

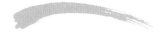

swings, and high blood pressure. Alternatively, slow and relaxed breathing calms our body, soothes our thoughts, helps regulate our emotions, improves digestion, and may decrease physical pain. In other words, with the practice of balanced breathing you can live your day feeling free, open, and balanced.

When practicing slow, deep breaths you allow yourself to move beyond survival and into a new state of being. Deep and relaxed breathing can lead to reduced tension and stress, a greater amount of energy, general well-being, and a connection to your own self. In short, with proper breathing you will be less neurotic.

If someone is breathing very rapidly and attempting to "think positively," it will likely yield little, if any, results. This is why in mental imagery and hypnosis the practitioner guides the client to take deep breaths through the nose and complete exhalations through the mouth. After this step, positive thoughts become a more natural experience.

Furthermore, thoughts are experiences! Ask yourself, what experience would you like to have right now in your own mind? Perhaps you want to go beyond survival and guide yourself into a more vital state of being. Start using your mind so your mind stops using you.

The idea of deep breathing is very much associated with the relationship between Lung Qi and Kidney Qi. Kidney Qi is responsible for "grasping" the Lung Qi. In other words, the Kidneys take in the life force of oxygen and use it to build Qi for proper functioning of the systems of the body. This can only be done with proper breathing. The Kidneys hold our Kidney Jing (see page 25), which is responsible for determining our constitution, reproductive functioning, growth, and aging process. Therefore, you may be prolonging your life with deep breaths. As a matter of fact, many yogis believe that we only have a certain amount of breaths. So remember, just breathe.

A Guide to Essential Oils

The following oils are used in the treatments in this book. You will discover how each one is classified, in terms of the different groups we learned about in Chapter 2, and find out how it is commonly used.

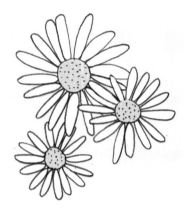

Roman Chamomile
(*Anthemis nobilis*)

CALMING, SOOTHING, AND SOFTENING

Roman chamomile (also known as English chamomile) is native to the United Kingdom. This cooling essential oil is a middle note, and it has a sweet scent. It has relaxing and calmative effects on the mind, heart, and digestive system, and is commonly used for its positive effects on nausea and indigestion. According to Chinese medicine, Roman chamomile has affinities to the Heart, Liver, and Spleen.

Obtained from flowers, this essential oil is calming to the mind, soothing to the nerves, and it can cool an upsurge of Yang energy, making it very beneficial for people who are quick to anger, short-tempered, harsh, or judgmental. Roman chamomile assists in soothing the Liver Qi (transforming agitation and irritability into calmness and smoothness) and clearing Heat and Fire from the Liver and Heart.

In terms of digestive disharmonies, this essential oil is beneficial for harmonizing the Liver and the Spleen, which means that it is always used in blends when the Liver (Wood) is overacting on the Spleen (Earth) (see page 109).

Here's a simple way to help you remember Roman chamomile's relationship with the Liver and Spleen: its flowers have white petals and a yellow center. Yellow is the color connected with the Spleen and the solar plexus chakra, which is very much associated with our ego, sense of self, and self-assertiveness. Therefore, Roman chamomile is a key oil to use when working on people who have a perfectionist, type-A personality, and for those people who aren't open to others' influence (in other words, people who have a Wood constitution, see pages 34–35). Floral oils are associated with opening to our vulnerabilities, but Roman chamomile's connection to the Liver means that it is especially good at helping people to improve the way they communicate with others, stopping them from being a tyrant.

Roman chamomile is closely related to the solar plexus chakra, so in most treatments the oil is placed on the Ren 12 point, which harmonizes and soothes the solar plexus.

Roman chamomile is commonly used in skincare creams to reduce inflammation.

Its cooling and calming nature makes it the ideal oil for all heat-related symptoms. This might be as straightforward as alleviating inflammation and pain from overuse and overstrain, such as tennis or golfer's elbow. However, Roman chamomile also works on the emotional heat we see with Liver Fire or Heart Fire. Liver Fire and Heart Fire are commonly considered separate Chinese medicine diagnoses, but they blend with each other. Wood engenders Fire, meaning that Liver engenders the Heart; and the Heart is specific to Fire, so whenever there is any kind of emotional agitation it affects both the Heart and the Liver. Roman chamomile can be beneficial for people who are quick to anger, irritable, or have violent tendencies, as well as for vertex headaches (a headache at the crown of the head).

Roman chamomile blends well with lavender, bergamot, lemongrass, and patchouli, to name just a few.

Level of Qi:
Ying

Fragrance note:
Middle

Part of the plant:
Flowers

Temperature:
Cooling

Meridian/organ:
Liver, Spleen, Heart

Element:
Wood, Fire, Earth

Blends well with:
Bergamot, geranium, lavender, peppermint, vetiver

Physical actions:
Reduces inflammation; clears Heat; calms the mind; soothes Liver Qi

Emotional actions:
Eases impatience and irritability; soothes the nerves and anger

Comparing Roman Chamomile with Rosemary

When learning about essential oils, it is helpful to compare oils with each other. A comparison that I like to make is between rosemary (see page 84) and Roman chamomile. These oils both are useful for disharmonies of the Liver and Spleen, but rosemary is warming and sends the Liver Qi upward, while Roman chamomile softens the Liver Qi, and soothes anger and irritability. Rosemary strongly promotes the movement of Qi; Roman chamomile quiets the Qi. In other words, rosemary promotes more expression, while Roman chamomile allows someone to accept what is.

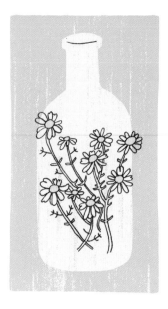

German Chamomile
(*Matricaria recutita*)

PEACEFUL, TRUSTING, AND ACCEPTING

German chamomile is native to Europe, but the essential oil is most commonly distilled in Egypt and Hungary and is often distilled in the United Kingdom. Many people have an aversion to the oil's very sweet scent; therefore it's wise to use a small amount the first time you work with German chamomile.

German chamomile oil can be a deep ocean-blue color. This blue color connects it to the Water element, which is responsible for cooling Heart Fire. German chamomile has the ability to cool, clear Heat, and induce calm. It can cool Fire that is being expressed on the physical level, such as boils, carbuncles, and burns, which are all examples of Heat in the body that is being released. It can also cool Fire that is being expressed on an emotional level, such as the expression of repressed anger, which is often connected to Liver and Heart Fire.

As with Roman chamomile (see page 56), any oils that can clear Heat are beneficial for painful joints. German and Roman chamomile are both particularly beneficial for pain around the elbow joint. Why? Because the Large Intestine 11 and Heart 3 acupressure points are both located around the elbow—both of these points clear Heat and can decrease inflammation. When using German chamomile for inflammation and pain around the elbow, I would always add frankincense to the blend.

Level of Qi:
Ying–Yuan

Fragrance note:
Middle–base

Part of the plant:
Flowers

Temperature:
Cooling

Meridian/organ:
Heart, Kidney

Element:
Water

Blends well with:
Bergamot, geranium, spikenard, ylang-ylang

Physical actions:
Reduces inflammation; cools Heat; soothes Liver and Heart Fire

Emotional actions:
Eases anger and impatience

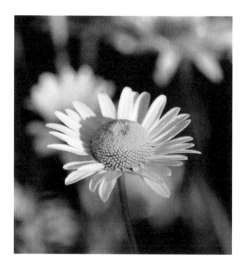

COMPARING ROMAN CHAMOMILE WITH GERMAN CHAMOMILE

	ROMAN CHAMOMILE	GERMAN CHAMOMILE
Part of Plant	Flower	Flower
Plant Characteristics	A perennial plant. It generally grows low to the ground, and can be used as ground-cover. The plant has hairy stems and its flowers have white petals and a yellow center.	A self-seeding plant that can grow taller than Roman chamomile. It has hairless stems. Its flowers are similar to Roman chamomile, but larger.
Organs and Meridians	Liver and Spleen	Heart and Kidney
Country of Distillation	United Kingdom and USA	Hungary and Germany
Oil Color	Water white or pale blue	Intense blue (due to chamazulene)
Scent	Diffuse, very sweet, fruity aroma	Heavy, sweet aroma
Element	Wood (and secondary Fire)	Fire and Water
Common Patterns	Liver Fire: insomnia, restlessness, expressions of anger, violent tendencies. Wood overacting on Earth: irritability with alternating constipation and diarrhea, pain in the sides of the ribs. Feeling emotionally stuck: PMS symptoms, acute breathlessness and anxiety "asthma." Beneficial for people with a type-A personality, goal-setters and goal-seekers who don't take the time needed to nourish themselves and to be nourished by others.	Heart Fire: skin eruptions, explosive anger, insomnia, restlessness, palpitations, joint pain that is worse with heat. May cool impulsive behavior for those who act out of passion and not reason.
Chakra	Solar plexus	Heart and throat

Level of Qi:
Yuan

Fragrance note:
Base

Part of the plant:
Resin

Temperature:
Cooling

Meridian/organ:
Lung, Heart, Kidney

Element:
Fire, Metal, Water

Blends well with:
Bergamot, geranium, lavender, lemongrass, peppermint, sweet marjoram

Physical actions:
Calms the mind; cools inflammation; reduces the appearance of scars; opens the chest

Emotional actions:
Eases grief; brings clarity to life situations

Frankincense

(*Boswellia carteri* and *Boswellia sacra*)

HEALER OF PHYSICAL AND EMOTIONAL WOUNDS

Commonly distilled in Oman and Somalia, frankincense is considered to be one of the most sacred of essential oils. It is often used for rituals and in incense. The Ancient Egyptians used frankincense to make insect repellents, perfumes, salves, and the eyeliner known as kohl.

Frankincense resin is obtained by slashing the bark of the boswellia tree: the milky white resin that the tree exudes in order to heal itself is later distilled to become the essential oil. This process provides us with the key to frankincense's ability to mend physical and emotional wounds. The oil is particularly effective for working with emotional wounds that have not been healed, and for letting go of the past.

Frankincense is associated with the Lung system, and it may be beneficial for chronic lung conditions. As you may remember from Chapter 2, the Lungs are connected with grief (see page 41), so frankincense can be used during times of prolonged grief or sadness, when those emotions are keeping a person from performing their responsibilities in the physical world. Frankincense can be blended with ravensara, tea tree, or Scots pine to strengthen the Lung Qi.

Frankincense is also paired with the Heart and the Kidney systems, which makes it an excellent choice for nervousness and fatigue. The oil carries the function to increase the depth of respiration and to calm the Shen (see page 27).

This cooling oil is very beneficial for alleviating inflammation and pain. It can be used by itself or blended with Roman chamomile, lavender, or geranium to assist its Heat-clearing abilities.

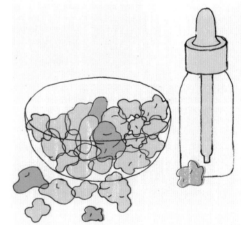

Ylang-ylang (*Cananga odorata*)

COOLING, UPLIFTING, CHARISMATIC, AND FLIRTATIOUS

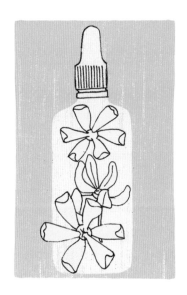

Ylang-ylang is obtained from the flowers of the cananga tree, which grows in Southeast Asia. The flowers have a sweet, sensual scent, and the name ylang-ylang means "flower of flowers." These days, most ylang-ylang essential oil is distilled in Madagascar.

The abundantly rich fragrance of ylang-ylang has made it popular as a perfume base for centuries. A very small amount of this sweet, concentrated essential oil goes a long way. The scent of ylang-ylang is so deep that it is extracted using a fractionated distillation method, which pulls out different layers of the multi-dimensional fragrance in stages. The initial distillation is called ylang-ylang extra, and this first-pass extraction is the most prized for perfumery, the most costly, and the sweetest. Further distillations are categorized as ylang-ylang I, ylang-ylang II, and ylang-ylang III. The scent becomes somewhat lighter with each of the later distillations, and each of these grades has its own distinct character. Sometimes a grade of oil called ylang-ylang complete can be found on the market, which is usually a blending of all four distillations, but may also be a full, uninterrupted distillation.

Like geranium (see page 77), ylang-ylang nourishes the Yin, calms the Shen (see page 27), moisturizes the skin, and it has been said to help hair with split ends. It is regarded as a strong aphrodisiac, and it is often used in women's perfume. In fact, it is a key scent in the famous Chanel No. 5.

The cananga tree (also known as the perfume tree) has yellow star-shaped flowers that tend to grow in clusters, and look as if they are intermingling. These characteristics allude to the oil's therapeutic uses. Ylang-ylang is known to bring out charisma, confidence, and sensuality. It can be beneficial for those who are inhibited about sexuality, flirtation, or showing their inner creativity to the world.

Ylang-ylang is primarily associated with the Heart, and it is very efficient at cooling Heart Fire and nourishing the Blood. The cooling nature of ylang-ylang makes it suitable to treat symptoms of restlessness, anxiety, general tension, insomnia, and irritability.

The very feminine nature of ylang-ylang means that it can balance out those people who have a type-A personality, and it can assist people to open up to receptivity and nourishment. I often use this oil for people who are not in a nourishing relationship. The oil blends well with jasmine and rose, both of which are also revered for their effects on the feminine.

Level of Qi:
Ying, Yuan

Fragrance note:
Middle, base

Part of the plant:
Flowers

Temperature:
Cooling

Meridian/organ:
Heart, Kidney

Element:
Fire, Water

Blends well with:
Blood orange, geranium, lavender, neroli, patchouli

Physical actions:
Eases insomnia; cools the Heart and Liver

Emotional actions:
Eases anxiety, irritability, restlessness, and tension; encourages the expression of creativity; dispels sexual inhibitions; promotes joy

Level of Qi:
Ying, Yuan

Fragrance note:
Middle, base

Part of the plant:
Flowers

Temperature:
Cooling

Meridian/organ:
Heart, Spleen

Element:
Fire, Earth

Blends well with:
Blood orange, lemongrass, patchouli, sweet fennel, ylang-ylang

Physical actions:
Calms the Shen; soothes the nerves; supports digestion

Emotional actions:
Eases anxiety, worry, and fear

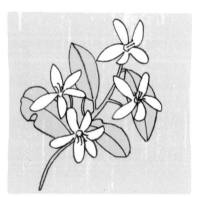

Neroli *(Citrus aurantium ssp. aurantium flos.)*

THE PRECIOUS PRESENT MOMENT

Neroli essential oil is derived from the flower blossoms of the bitter orange tree, which grows around the Mediterranean. The tree also yields an essential oil from its peel, leaves, and twigs, which is known as petitgrain.

Neroli is one of the most expensive essential oils. It takes about 1,000 lb (450 kg) of flowers to make just 1 lb (0.5 kg) of oil. Ideally, the essential oil is extracted through steam distillation of the flowers in order to preserve the delicate composition of neroli oil. Much less care is required in the distillation process for petitgrain.

Due to the high cost of production, it is not uncommon to find that neroli oil has been co-distilled with petitgrain oil. A legitimate supplier will label adulterated oil as "neroli petitgrain" or "petitgrain sur le fleurs," which means they are being honest about the fact that the oil is not 100 percent neroli.

Neroli is beneficial for physical, emotional, and mental ailments. Of all the floral oils, neroli is the most grounding and stabilizing. It can assist people in being present, especially when they are ready to make a commitment to improving their physical health, and it also works to align the mind and body. No floral oil is more associated with the will and with "staying the course" than neroli.

In Chinese medicine, neroli is associated with the Spleen and Heart. This makes it an integral oil to use when there are physical ailments such as digestive disorders stemming from anxiety and/or fear. Neroli is one of the best oils for people who have a history of nervousness and anxiety that leads to digestive troubles.

Uniquely among the floral oils, neroli has the ability to tonify the Spleen. This ability to act on an emotional or psychological level means that neroli is beneficial for people who have a Spleen Qi deficiency, especially issues with boundaries. Such people often have noticeable broken capillaries or spider veins. Neroli is very beneficial for people who give love and help to others as a way to fill something that is lacking in their own lives, rather than out of a sense of good will.

Neroli tonifies the Heart Qi and Spleen Qi, and as such it will aid with discernment and the withholding of giving too much of oneself. In terms of the Heart, neroli is one of the best oils to use when there is anxiety. It is known to regulate the rhythm of the heart, and can be used for those with chronic anxiety, insomnia, and fear.

Bergamot (*Citrus bergamia*)

SOOTHING, UPLIFTING, AND SOFTENING

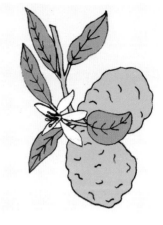

This essential oil is obtained from the peel of the bergamot tree's fruit. Bergamot oil is naturally cooling. It is wonderful for uplifting one's mood, and I often recommend diffusing it in stressful office environments. Bergamot is known to be the softest of the citruses, and it tends to blend well with most other oils.

My clients just love the uplifting and relaxing effect of bergamot. Of all the citrus oils, bergamot is the one used most frequently in my practice. Quite often when I am treating a client in the prone position, I will put a drop of bergamot on a tissue and place it under the massage table headrest so the client can enjoy the aroma throughout the session.

Bergamot oil is a top note. It is best used in a blend with *Eucalyptus radiata*, peppermint, and tea tree to Release the Exterior (see page 14). It is also appropriate to use for Wind-Heat (see page 88) if the person has underlying Qi stagnation with symptoms of irritability and frustration.

Bergamot can be used in blends to soothe anxiety and promote the movement of Liver Qi. Often it is blended with lavender and Roman chamomile when there is emotional stress causing digestive issues.

Bergamot's greenish color gives us a clue that it is beneficial for the Liver Qi—the Liver is associated with the Wood element and the color green (see page 33). And for those who are interested in the chakras, bergamot is certainly going to be beneficial for the heart chakra, which is also associated with the color green.

Bergamot can assist with grief when it is blended with frankincense and either ravensara or tea tree. Although these blends can help to uplift one's spirits when moving through the grieving process, by no means are they intended to take the place of a qualified therapist. They should be used in conjunction with professional guidance.

CAUTION: Using bergamot

Bergamot can cause photosensitivity. Always dilute the essential oil with a base oil, at a maximum 0.4 percent concentration (see dilution chart on page 51), which is equivalent to 1 drop in 2 teaspoons (10 ml) base oil.

Be very careful when transferring bergamot and other citrus oils to a blending bottle. The oil is very thin and flows quickly, so you will only need to tilt the bottle a little before the oil drips out.

Level of Qi:
Wei

Fragrance note:
Top

Part of the plant:
Peel

Temperature:
Cooling

Meridian/organ:
Lung, Liver, Stomach

Element:
Wood, Fire

Blends well with:
Most oils, particularly German and Roman chamomile, lavender, peppermint, spikenard

Physical actions:
Dispels Wind-Heat; Releases the Exterior; moves Liver Qi

Emotional actions:
Refreshes; uplifts; eases irritability, frustration, and grief

Level of Qi:
Wei

Fragrance note:
Top

Part of the plant:
Peel

Temperature:
Cooling

Meridian/organ:
Lung, Heart, Stomach,
Spleen

Element:
Fire, Earth

Blends well with:
Lemon, neroli, patchouli

Physical actions:
Dispels Wind-Heat

Emotional actions:
Brightens the mood;
refreshes; uplifts

Blood Orange (*Citrus sinensis*)

JOYFUL, UPBEAT, AND INNOCENT

Blood orange essential oil is cooling, refreshing, and uplifting. It is a variant of sweet orange (sometimes just called orange), and it has a more complex smell. The overall personality of blood orange is happy. It is a beautiful oil to use to uplift one's spirits, though its effects don't last long.

Derived from citrus peel, this oil is beneficial in blends to Release the Exterior (see page 14) due to Wind-Heat (see page 88). However, it is most often added to blends to assist other essential oils. Blood orange has an affinity with the Lungs and the Wei Qi (see page 14), and it is also associated with the Stomach, Spleen, and Heart.

A four percent concentration (see dilution chart on page 51) is a safe dermal application for blood orange. It is best to store the oil in a refrigerator as it can oxidize quickly and turn rancid.

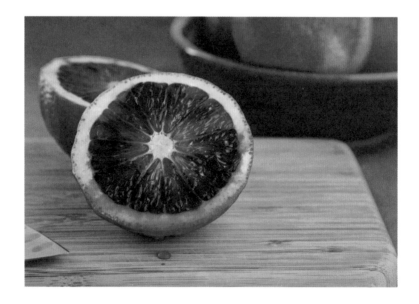

Lemongrass *(Cymbopogon citratus)*

WARMING, UPLIFTING, REFRESHING, AND INVIGORATING

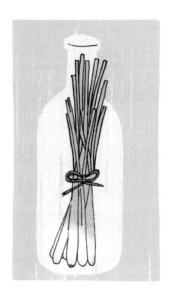

Lemongrass is a warming, aromatic essential oil with a fresh and lemony scent. Known as the connective tissue or tendinomusclar oil, lemongrass promotes the movement of Qi in our musculoskeletal system. It is associated with Liver and Gall Bladder meridians.

Lemongrass is the premier oil for alleviating hip and leg pain by promoting the movement of Qi. When the Liver Qi ceases to rise upward, it descends and causes stagnation. As a Chinese medicine saying goes, "If there is no free flow, there is pain." Symbolically, the leg is associated with moving forward in life. This is directly in parallel with the function of promoting the free flow of Qi.

Lemongrass benefits digestion and emotional stagnation. Much like rosemary (see page 84), it has an assertive nature, and it is used to strengthen our solar plexus and help us to maintain boundaries. Also like rosemary, lemongrass is often used for symptoms when the Liver (Wood) is overacting on the Spleen (Earth) (see page 109). Lemongrass can be used with Roman chamomile, lavender, and peppermint to promote the movement of Liver Qi and to harmonize the Liver and Spleen.

Lemongrass oil is yellowish in color—the color of the Spleen. Lemongrass revives the Spleen, and can aid it in transforming Dampness (see page 39). Lemongrass is an integral choice for a Spleen Qi deficiency with symptoms of heaviness and weak muscles. It can be used to strengthen weak or flaccid muscles, and to alleviate heaviness. The oil can be blended with peppermint and rosemary to relieve sluggishness, or with ginger to warm the muscles. Lemongrass is also psychologically uplifting.

CAUTION: Using lemongrass

Most oils should not be used directly on the skin unless they have been diluted (see page 51). This is particularly true for lemongrass oil, which can irritate the skin due to its high citral content.

Level of Qi:
Ying

Fragrance note:
Middle

Part of the plant:
Grass

Temperature:
Warming

Meridian/organ:
Liver, Spleen, Gall Bladder

Element:
Wood, Earth

Blends well with:
Lavender, orange, Roman chamomile, rosemary, vetiver

Physical actions:
Eases fatigue and muscle and joint pain that is worse with cold (especially hip pain); supports digestion; revives the Spleen

Emotional actions:
Eases melancholy; uplifts

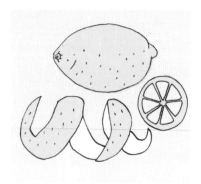

Lemon (*Citrus limon*)

CLEAN, ZESTY, AND INVIGORATING

Lemon has a clean, zesty, and invigorating aroma. It is a cooling top note, and as it is high in antibacterial and astringent functions, it is often used in blends for common colds and digestion.

Lemon is a great choice to diffuse in a room for its uplifting capability and ability to stimulate the mind and help focus. Try diffusing with *Eucalyptus radiata* or rosemary for this purpose. Due to its strong antibacterial function, lemon is also often used in house cleaners.

Lemon can be either cold pressed or steam distilled. If it is cold pressed it can be phototoxic (that is, it makes skin sensitive to light), like bergamot, but it will be fine if it is steam distilled. However, cold pressed lemon oil has the best aroma.

Please note that lemon is not related to lemongrass or lemon balm (*Melissa officinalis*).

Level of Qi:
Wei

Fragrance note:
Top

Part of the plant:
Peel

Temperature:
Cooling

Meridian/organ:
Lung, Spleen, Liver

Element:
Wood, Earth, Metal

Blends well with:
Other citruses, frankincense, neroli, eucalyptus, geranium, cypress

Physical actions:
Refreshes; Releases the Exterior; assists in strengthening the Spleen and alleviating dampness and feelings of sluggishness

Emotional actions:
Uplifts; beneficial for those that worry or lack focus

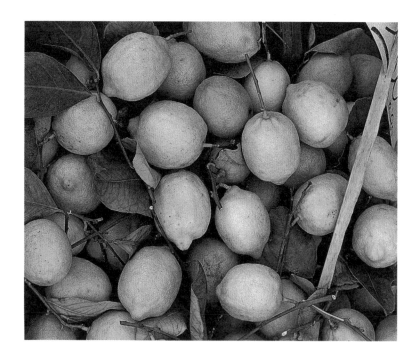

Peppermint (*Mentha × piperata*)

RELEASES THE EXTERIOR AND PROMOTES QI

Peppermint is one of the most esteemed essential oils. It awakens the senses and refreshes the mind. Peppermint has a wide array of therapeutic functions that are related to the upper body and the digestive system. Common conditions that peppermint treats include sinus congestion, heavy-headedness, mental fatigue, headaches, neck pain, nausea, and irritability.

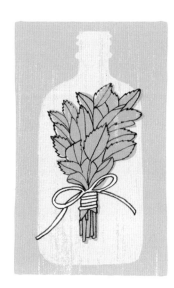

Peppermint has an affinity with the Lungs and Liver, so it's not surprising that two major TCM functions of peppermint oil are Releasing the Exterior (see page 14) and the promotion of Liver Qi.

Neck pain is one of the most common ailments that I see in my practice. Peppermint has analgesic properties and is often used for neck pain. The philosophy of Chinese medicine can bring about a deeper understanding of the causes of pain and the correct treatment strategies. For example, neck pain can be a symptom of the common cold (Wind-Heat or Wind-Cold) (see page 88), Qi stagnation, or Blood deficiency. Peppermint should be used to treat neck pain due to the common cold or Qi stagnation, but it is not indicated for neck pain due to Blood deficiency, which should be treated with Roman chamomile and palmarosa.

Wind is naturally Yang, which means that it will affect the upper and the outer areas of the body. There are two types of Wind (see page 37): external wind and internal wind. External wind is a major causative factor of illness. If the External Wind is not treated, it is likely that the pathogen will make its way into the interior and cause more serious illness. Although External Wind is usually associated with literal wind, we can understand External Wind to mean changes that we are going through in life. These changes can be a real "Pain in the Neck." Therefore, it is essential to Release the Exterior, and peppermint does just that.

Level of Qi:
Wei

Fragrance note:
Top–middle

Part of the plant:
Leaves

Temperature:
Cooling

Meridian/organ:
Lung, Liver

Element:
Wood, Metal

Blends well with:
Basil, *Eucalyptus globulus*, *Eucalyptus radiata*, frankincense, lavender, Roman chamomile, rosemary

Physical actions:
Dispels Wind-Heat; eases neck pain, sinus congestion, nausea, temporal headaches, heavy-headedness, and mental fatigue; Releases the Exterior; promotes Liver Qi

Emotional actions:
Uplifts; awakens; eases irritability and frustration

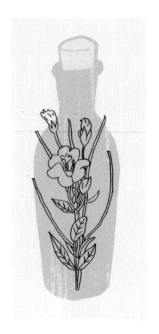

Palmarosa (*Cymbopogon martini*)

SOOTHING AND PEACEFUL

Palmarosa essential oil is distilled from grass, yet its cooling, calming, and nourishing actions are more similar to those of a floral oil.

Palmarosa is a very adaptable essential oil, and it has many functions. It can be used to nourish the Yin, calm the Shen (see page 27), and Release the Exterior (see page 14). Palmarosa is particularly beneficial to those who are new to holistic healing, as it aids in feelings of calmness and openness. It also nourishes the skin, and for this reason it is used in many skincare creams.

In Western terms, palmarosa is known to be high in antiviral properties, and it can be used in cases of boils and for toxic heat on the skin. This is, of course, beyond the scope of this book, but I've mentioned it to demonstrate the extent to which essential oils can be used for healing.

Palmarosa is an ideal choice for any form of anxiety. We all experience anxiety at one time or another. Common symptoms may include palpitations, lack of focus, insomnia, nervousness, fear, and worry. When we examine these symptoms, we can see that many of them are related to concerns about what may happen in the future. Palmarosa is a great remedy that allows us to be relaxed and to focus on the present moment.

Level of Qi:
Wei, Ying

Fragrance note:
Top–middle

Part of the plant:
Grass

Temperature:
Cooling

Meridian/organ:
Lung, Pericardium

Element:
Fire

Blends well with:
German and Roman chamomile, geranium, lavender, ylang-ylang

Physical actions:
Nourishes the skin; soothes the nerves; calms the Shen

Emotional actions:
Eases anxiety and nervousness

Cardamom (*Elettaria cardamomum*)

A FRAGRANT AWAKENING

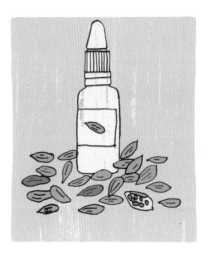

Cardamom is a strongly aromatic spice that is used in a multitude of dishes, both sweet and savory. Its powerful acrid action cuts through stagnation, which is why the spice is commonly added to heavy dishes containing sugar, dairy, or meat.

The use of this spice dates back over 4,000 years. The Ancient Egyptians used cardamom in medicated salves and for religious rites, while the Ancient Greeks prized cardamom for its pleasant scent, using it to create perfumes and oils for body hygiene.

As far as Chinese medicine is concerned, cardamom is mostly used to aid digestion, aromatically open the orifices, and transform Dampness (see page 39). The Spleen-Stomach network (see page 108) governs smooth digestion and the extraction of nutrients from food to create energy. If this process is impaired due to an imbalanced diet, stress, or other trigger, the Spleen-Stomach becomes inefficient. The digestive system then suffers a chronic level of inflammation and poor cell-waste metabolism. This state is often categorized as Dampness, and it contributes not only to digestive sluggishness but also decreased mental clarity. Cardamom can be blended with lemon to open the orifices and revive the Spleen.

Level of Qi:
Ying

Fragrance note:
Middle

Part of the plant:
Seeds

Temperature:
Warming

Meridian/organ:
Lung, Spleen, Kidney

Element:
Earth, Metal

Blends well with:
Orange, patchouli,
sweet fennel

Physical actions:
Supports digestion;
aromatically opens
the orifices

Emotional actions:
Eases worry

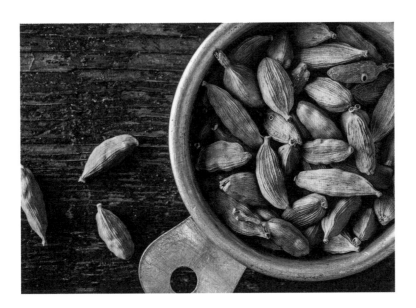

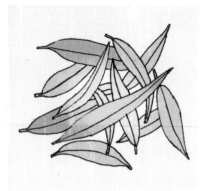

Eucalyptus (*Eucalyptus globulus*)

OPENING, CLEARING, AND EXPANDING

Eucalyptus globulus (also known as the Tasmanian blue gum) is an evergreen tree that is native to Australia. Its leaves and branches produce a warming essential oil that has a wide array of functions, including Releasing the Exterior for Wind-Cold (see page 88), transforming Cold Phlegm (phlegm that is clear) in the Lungs, alleviating pain in the upper body, and benefiting pain associated with arthritis.

Just like *Eucalyptus radiata* (see page opposite), *Eucalyptus globulus* is rich in 1,8 cineole (see page 85), which means that it is high in antibacterial and antiviral properties. However, one major difference between these two oils is that *Eucalyptus globulus* is warming, whereas *Eucalyptus radiata* is cooling.

Eucalyptus globulus's warming nature makes it an ideal choice for the symptoms of Wind-Cold, and to decongest the lungs in cases of Cold Phlegm. In fact, it is frequently used in lozenges for sore throats and in cough syrups as an expectorant. This essential oil can be blended with Scots pine, *Eucalyptus radiata*, and tea tree.

Eucalyptus globulus is also the premier oil for Wind-Damp Cold, more commonly known in Western medicine as arthritis. For this purpose, it can be blended with vetiver, ginger, and frankincense.

Level of Qi:
Wei, Ying

Fragrance note:
Top, middle

Part of the plant:
Leaves and branches

Temperature:
Warming

Meridian/organ:
Lung

Element:
Metal

Blends well with:
Basil, lemongrass, peppermint, rosemary, sweet marjoram

Physical actions:
Dispels Wind-Cold; eases chest congestion, pain in the upper body, and pain associated with arthritis

Emotional actions:
Allows for space when feeling emotionally suffocated

CAUTION: Using *Eucalyptus globulus*

Eucalyptus globulus has a high 1,8 cineole content and should be used with caution. It is contraindicated for direct inhalation by children under ten[1]. In a room diffuser, it is probably too diluted to be a bother to small children.

Eucalyptus globulus is not recommended for steam inhalations as it can irritate the throat and sinuses—instead, use peppermint or *Eucalyptus radiata* for a steam inhalation to decongest the sinuses.

Eucalyptus (*Eucalptus radiata*)

COOLING, UPLIFTING, AND QUICKENING

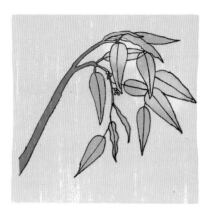

Eucalyptus radiata (commonly known as narrow-leaved peppermint) is native to Australia. Its essential oil is often considered to have the most pleasant aroma of all the eucalyptus oils used in aromatherapy.

Eucalyptus radiata is praised for its ability to alleviate the symptoms of the common cold due to its antibacterial and antiviral nature. In Western terms, this is due to its high content of 1,8 cineole (see page 85). With its aromatically fresh, clean, and opening scent and its cooling nature, *Eucalyptus radiata* is often the go-to oil when there are symptoms of Wind-Heat (see page 88). It is especially beneficial for a runny nose or nasal congestion, and it is an exceptional expectorant.

Eucalyptus radiata has uplifting and quickening qualities, and it is energizing to those who feel heavy-headed or sluggish. Dampness (see page 39) and heaviness are the result of Spleen Qi deficiency and poor dietary habits. Spleen Qi deficiency is often the cause of chest congestion, so if we want to truly treat sluggishness and chest congestion then we need to support the actions of *Eucalyptus radiata* with oils that tonify the Lung Qi and Spleen Qi, such as rosemary.

Level of Qi:
Wei

Fragrance note:
Top

Part of the plant:
Leaves

Temperature:
Cooling

Meridian/organ:
Lung

Element:
Metal

Blends well with:
Basil, *Eucalyptus globulus*, frankincense, peppermint, rosemary

Physical actions:
Dispels Wind-Heat; eases sinus congestion and upper body aches

Emotional actions:
Uplifts

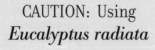

CAUTION: Using *Eucalyptus radiata*

Eucalyptus radiata has a high 1,8 cineole content and should be used with caution. It is contraindicated for children under ten[2].

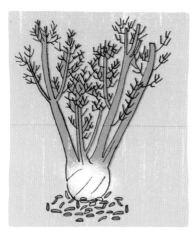

Sweet Fennel (*Foeniculum vulgare*)

WARMING, TRANSFORMING, AND COURAGEOUS

Sweet fennel essential oil is distilled from seeds. This warming and nourishing oil has a spicy and fragrant aroma that is similar to anise or licorice. Like ginger (see page 83), sweet fennel is commonly used to aid digestion due to its ability to tonify the Kidney Qi (the body's energy storehouse) and the Spleen Qi (responsible for the digestive system and digestive functions).

Sweet fennel is especially beneficial when there is a bodily sensation of sluggishness and Dampness (see page 39). One of the key symptoms of Dampness is heaviness and fatigue in the limbs. Sweet fennel has the function to tonify the Yang (associated with courage and stamina), and it can transform Dampness. In fact, the warriors of ancient Rome believed that eating fennel would make them strong and ready for fighting.

Sweet fennel seeds are commonly served after dairy-laden Indian food as they aid in the digestion of heavy, Damp food. Sweet fennel also warms the center, and it has a connection to the Du meridian that runs along the spine.

Level of Qi:
Ying

Fragrance note:
Middle

Part of the plant:
Seeds

Temperature:
Warming

Meridian/organ:
Lung, Spleen, Kidney

Element:
Earth, Metal, Water

Blends well with:
Blood orange, cardamom, lemongrass, patchouli

Physical actions:
Supports digestion; warms the Spleen

Emotional actions:
Eases fear

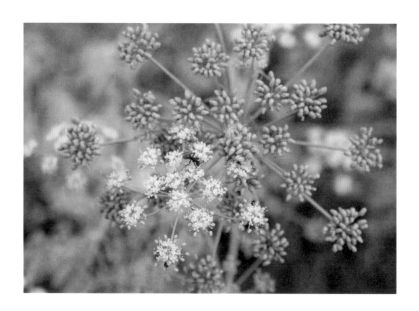

Lavender (*Lavandula angustifolia*)

GENTLY MOVING, UPLIFTING, AND RELAXING

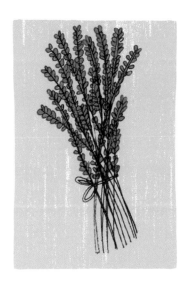

Lavender is one of the most beloved and well-used essential oils. It has an opening, soothing, and cooling nature, and it is famous for its ability to calm the nerves, relax the mind, and gently move the Qi, making it beneficial for just about anyone.

Lavender's most popular use is as a relaxant. Like bergamot (see page 63), it blends well with most oils. It can lift blends that are a bit heavy, and it can soften blends that are too ascending or warming.

This oil has the ability to open the chest, calm the Shen (see page 27), and cool Liver and Heart Fire. It also promotes the movement of Qi in the chest, and can be blended with *Eucalyptus radiata*, *Eucalyptus globulus*, and ravensara to expel phlegm.

Lavender aids in Releasing the Exterior (see page 14), which mean that it can be blended with other oils with that function to address the symptoms of Wind-Heat or Wind-Cold (see page 88). However, lavender is best used when there are also underlying symptoms of Liver Qi stagnation.

Lavender is also associated with moving blocked emotional Qi. Since lavender oil is distilled from flowers, it is able to open the chest in a way that will allow someone to begin to express their gentler side, or to share things that have been festering for some time. Often lavender is blended with peppermint for this purpose. Both of these oils have affinities with the Lungs and Liver, and they aid in promoting the movement of Qi in the chest.

One of lavender's most important functions is to ensure that the energy of the Liver moves smoothly. Lavender is key when there are symptoms of Qi stagnation such as acute irritability, frequent sighing, pain in the side of the ribs, and bloating. Lavender is the oil that you should carry with you throughout the day in order to aid in moving mild daily irritations and frustrations. One great way to use the oil for this purpose is to diffuse it in a stressful workplace.

Lavender can be blended with lemongrass and sweet marjoram for Qi stagnation in the Gall Bladder meridian, with symptoms of pain in the buttocks that travels along the Gall Bladder meridian of the leg.

The body is always searching for balance, so a Qi stagnation that is left untreated will eventually erupt. (Just imagine, for example, covering a pot of boiling water with a lid—eventually it is going to boil over.) This eruption can be thought of as Liver Fire (see page 57). Lavender and Roman chamomile are often blended to cool and calm Liver Qi, cool an excessive expression of anger, or calm the Shen.

Level of Qi:
Wei

Fragrance note:
Top

Part of the plant:
Flowers

Temperature:
Cooling

Meridian/organ:
Lung, Liver, Heart

Element:
Wood, Fire

Blends well with:
Bergamot, geranium, palmarosa, peppermint, Roman chamomile

Physical actions:
Soothes the nerves; calms the Shen; opens the chest; cools Fire; moves Liver Qi

Emotional actions:
Eases grief; aids the expression of creativity

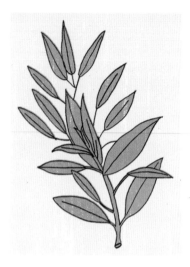

Tea Tree (*Melaleuca alternifolia*)

STRENGTHENING, PROTECTIVE, AND BOLD

Tea tree is one of the best-known essential oils. It is high in antibacterial qualities, and it is commonly found in soaps, toothpaste, and a variety of other household products. Tea tree has a cool, clean, fresh, and medicinal scent.

Recognized as a broad-spectrum antibacterial, antiviral, and antifungal oil, tea tree has a long history of medicinal use. Indigenous Australian peoples first discovered tea tree's antiseptic qualities, using it to heal cuts and bruises. Tea tree oil can be used for acne, athlete's foot, and other fungal and bacterial infections. Tea tree is also beneficial for the muscle aches and pains associated with the flu, Qi stagnation in the upper body, and lower back pain due to a Kidney Qi deficiency.

As a middle note, tea tree oil has the ability to tonify the Lung Qi, making it ideal for a person who has frequent common colds, shortness of breath, a persistent cough, perhaps a soft voice with a dislike of speaking, upper body edema, and so on.

Tea tree has an affinity with not only the Lungs but also the Kidneys, and it is beneficial in assisting the Kidneys to "grasp" the Lung Qi (see page 54). Tea tree can be combined with Scots pine for a general Lung Qi deficiency or a dual deficiency of the Lungs and Kidneys. Symptoms of a dual deficiency of the Lungs and Kidneys are shortness of breath, wheezing, spontaneous sweating, lower back pain, fatigue, copious clear urination, and low libido.

Since both tea tree and Scots pine (see page 80) are associated with the Lungs and the Kidneys, they are a good combination to use when treating people who have breathing difficulties, such as asthma, or muscle aches and pains. Tea tree and Scots pine can be used with a compress for lower back pain due to Kidney Qi deficiency with accompanying symptoms of shortness of breath, lassitude, frequent urination, and knee and ankle pain.

A simple practical application that is beneficial for sore throats is to gargle with one drop of tea tree oil diluted in ⅓ cup (2½ fl oz/75 ml) water on the onset of throat pain.

Level of Qi:
Ying

Fragrance note:
Middle

Part of the plant:
Leaves

Temperature:
Cooling

Meridian/organ:
Lung, Kidney

Element:
Metal, Water

Blends well with:
Eucalyptus globulus,
Eucalyptus radiata,
frankincense, peppermint,
Scots pine

Physical actions:
Tonifies the Lung Qi; eases muscle aches and pains, particularly back pain; treats acne, athlete's foot, and other fungal and bacterial infections

Emotional actions:
Eases grief and fear

Basil (*Ocimum basilicum*)

WARMING, INVIGORATING, AND FOCUSING TO THE MIND

Basil (also known as sweet basil or French basil) has an uplifting and very aromatically open scent. Often used in Mediterranean cooking, this essential oil is distilled from the plant's leaves and flowering tops.

Basil's warming nature makes it one of the best oils to use for the symptoms of Wind-Cold (see page 88) and to support Wei Qi (see page 14). Basil can be blended with ravensara, tea tree, or rosemary in order to support both these functions.

Just like peppermint (see page 67), basil can loosen neck pain, alleviate sinus congestion, and help improve alertness. However, due to its warming nature, basil is most suitable for neck pain that is worse when it is cold and congestion with white or clear phlegm. Basil also tonifies the Yang and warms the Spleen, which means that it is an efficient oil to use for the symptoms of constipation.

There are many different chemotypes (see page 85) of basil, notably estragole and linalool. Exotic basil (the estragole chemotype) is the most hazardous. Sweet basil (the linalool chemotype) is the safest basil essential oil to use.

Level of Qi:
Wei, Ying

Fragrance note:
Top

Part of the plant:
Leaves and flowers

Temperature:
Warming

Meridian/organ:
Lungs, Spleen, Stomach

Element:
Earth, Metal

Blends well with:
Eucalyptus globulus,
Eucalyptus radiata,
lemongrass, peppermint,
rosemary

Physical actions:
Dispels Wind-Cold; eases upper body pain, nasal congestion, and constipation; tonifies the Yang; warms the Spleen

Emotional actions:
Promotes confidence

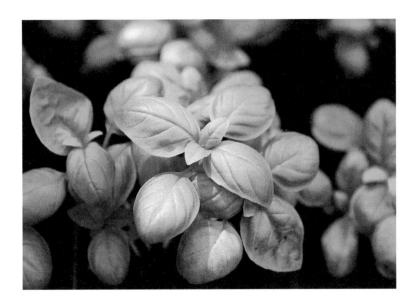

Level of Qi:
Yuan

Fragrance note:
Base

Part of the plant:
Roots

Temperature:
Cooling

Meridian/organ:
Heart, Pericardium,
Liver, Kidney

Element:
Water

Blends well with:
Bergamot, German
chamomile

Physical actions:
Descends Yang rising;
eases insomnia

Emotional actions:
Eases the feeling of being
scattered or unrooted;
promotes a connection to
deepest parts of your self

Spikenard
(*Nardostachys jatamansi*)

INWARD SANCTUARY

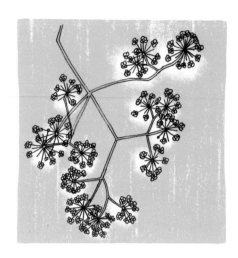

Spikenard (also known as false valerian root or simply as nard) is native to the Himalayas. The word "spikenard" in Hebrew is *nard*, which means "light." In ancient times, spikenard was one of the most expensive and sacred of essential oils. It is referenced several times in the Bible, and it is mentioned, along with myrrh and cinnamon, in King Solomon's Song of Songs.

Spikenard has a deep, heavy, musky scent. Most people find this scent to be overwhelming, and to have a sinking quality. The oil has an inward direction, which makes it beneficial for the symptoms associated with Fire, such as insomnia, certain kinds of headaches, and emotional agitation. Spikenard is especially beneficial during times of uncertainty, helping us to pull our energy inward and stay rooted.

Spikenard is associated with the Pericardium, Heart, Liver, and Kidneys. In terms of Chinese medicine, it is one of the best oils to use to sedate Liver Yang rising and to cool Heart Fire. Spikenard is considered one of the most sedative of all essential oils.

Like vetiver (see page 86), spikenard has an affinity with the lower aspects of the body, and it can be used to instil deep relaxation and calmness. Specific acupressure points that relate to spikenard are Kidney 1, Du 14, and Ren 4. It is also related to the sacral area (the base of the spine) and the soles of the feet.

Spikenard blends well with geranium, bergamot, and lavender, which are all calming oils that will uplift some of spikenard's downward direction.

CAUTION: Using spikenard

Spikenard should not be used to treat exterior conditions (see page 14) such as the common cold. This is because the oil's downward direction can draw pathogens inward.

Geranium (*Perlagonium graveolens*)

GRACEFUL, LOVING, AND KIND

The aroma of geranium is soft and mothering. The essential oil is distilled from the stems, velvety leaves, and flowers of the geranium plant, but most of the therapeutic properties come from the leaves. The oil is highly regarded in skincare products as it has the ability not only to soothe dry skin but also to hydrate it—making it a true skin balancer.

The geranium plant's leaves are soft and velvety, which gives us a clue to the oil's soft and calming ways. Another clue about this oil's nature is that the leaves hold water when it rains. Water is Yin, and it is equated to nourishment, so it should come as no surprise that this oil is also nourishing to the Yin.

Geranium's antifungal and antibacterial qualities mean that it has long been used in the treatment of fungal infections, such as athlete's foot, and eczema. It can also be used as an insect repellent, or to alleviate itching. All of the above are great ways to use geranium, but it is the oil's effect on the Heart and the Shen (see page 27) that carry its greatest attributes.

Geranium is very much connected to our Heart, Liver, and Kidneys. The oil can assist in forgiveness and opening up to new beginnings. In other words, it aids in opening up our Heart center and assists in the feelings of calmness and grace, giving us a sense of space. The spirit of geranium is that of a loving mother. Geranium can assist us when we are moving through life's changes, allowing us the space and peace to accept them. It may be beneficial to blend geranium with *Rosmarinus officinalis* ct. verbenone (see page 85) to aid in tonifying the Heart Qi. For as much as we need grace, love, and kindness to heal, we also need strength and fortitude.

Geranium is associated with nourishing the Yin and clearing Heat, and it is certainly a premier choice to cool and calm anxiety and restlessness.

As geranium opens the Heart, it can be used with lavender to increase intimate communication with yourself or your partner. In other words, it can help us open ourselves up to speak honestly, and it may allow those who need to be in control of relationships to be more yielding and accommodating.

Level of Qi:
Wei, Ying

Fragrance note:
Top, middle

Part of the plant:
Leaves, stalks, and flowers

Temperature:
Cooling

Meridian/organ:
Lung, Heart, Kidney, Liver

Element:
Fire, Water

Blends well with:
Bergamot, lavender, sandalwood, ylang-ylang

Physical actions:
Nourishes the skin; soothes the nerves; calms the Shen

Emotional actions:
Eases anxiety, restlessness, nervousness, and fear of communicating

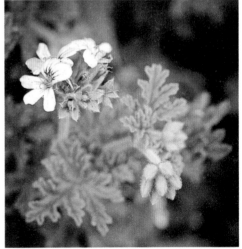

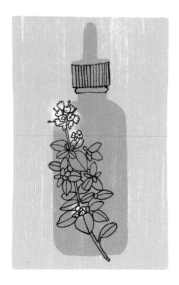

Level of Qi:
Wei, Ying

Fragrance note:
Top, middle

Part of the plant:
Leaves

Temperature:
Cooling and warming

Meridian/organ:
Lung, Liver

Element:
Wood, Fire

Blends well with:
Eucalyptus radiata,
frankincense, lavender,
lemongrass, ravensara,
tea tree

Physical actions:
Calms the Shen; eases
insomnia and muscle and
joint pain (particularly pain in
the neck, shoulder, and hips)

Emotional actions:
Eases anxiety

Sweet Marjoram (*Origanum majorana*)

A MUSCLE RELAXER

Sweet marjoram's Latin name is derived from the Greek words "oros" and "garnos," which can be translated as "joy of the mountains."

This essential oil is treasured for its cooling functions for the mind and spirit, yet it is also considered to be warming for its softening and pain relieving qualities on our muscles. It can be used as an analgesic for all muscle aches and discomfort, but it is particularly beneficial for pain in the muscles associated with the Gall Bladder meridian, and the muscles of the neck, shoulders, and hips. In fact, quite often when there is hip pain there is also pain in the neck and shoulders, and vice versa. For neck and shoulder pain, sweet marjoram can be blended with peppermint and *Eucalyptus radiata* or *Eucalyptus globulus*; and for hip pain it can be blended with lemongrass and *Eucalyptus globulus*.

According to Chinese medicine, the major functions of sweet marjoram include Releasing the Exterior (see page 14), promoting the movement of Qi, descending the Yang, and calming the Shen (see page 27).

Most often, when we speak about Releasing the Exterior, we are referring to the common cold, and Sweet marjoram can be used for Wind-Heat or Wind-Cold (see page 88), particularly when there are muscle aches and pains. The muscles are exterior in relationship to the organs, and the physical awareness of muscle pain is on the conscious level, which is why many oils that Release the Exterior also alleviate pain.

A common reason for pain in the neck and shoulders is Liver Yang Rising, most often caused by emotions and stress that rise to the surface but are not fully expressed outward. When this happens, the emotions and stress gets stuck or trapped in the upper shoulder area, as well as the jaw. Yang rising is quite common when there are stresses caused by relationships issues or work. Other symptoms common to Yang rising include headaches, insomnia, anger, dizziness, and pain in the neck, shoulders, and jaw. Sweet marjoram has the function to descend the Yang. Interestingly, this function correlates with the use of sweet marjoram to promote celibacy: it is considered an anaphrodisiac.

Sweet marjoram also aids in stress relief, calms the Shen, and relaxes the nerves. In addition to the oil's affinity with the upper back and hip muscles, it can also be used to relax muscles after a workout.

Patchouli (*Pogostemon cablin*)

SENSUOUS, MYSTERIOUS, AND NOURISHING

Patchouli essential oil has a rich, earthy, mysterious, and—to some—sensual scent. Once experienced, it is never forgotten. Patchouli is a base note, and it is beloved for its functions on many systems of the body. It has its main effects on the Heart, Spleen, and Stomach.

Patchouli is often associated with the free-loving hippie and New-Age movements of the 1960s, though its use as a medicinal plant dates back to Ancient Egypt. The patchouli plant is native to tropical regions of Asia, where it thrives in the damp environment and grows well during the rainy seasons.

Commonly grown in domestic gardens across Asia, the patchouli plant is used as a remedy for indigestion, nausea, diarrhea, food poisoning, and parasitism. In Chinese herbology, the leaves are used to combat patterns of Dampness (see page 39), when the Spleen-Stomach system is weakened or overwhelmed by poor diet, spoiled food, unclean water, or hot and damp weather. Patchouli has strong antifungal, antiviral, and antimicrobial properties, and it is often used to make incense, perfume, soaps, and cosmetics.

In terms of Chinese medicine, patchouli can calm the Shen (see page 27), clear Heat, harmonize the Spleen and Stomach, transform Dampness, and build Blood. In addition to its traditional Chinese medicine functions, patchouli can also be used as an aphrodisiac, and to heal minor skin irritations.

Patchouli can instil a deep sense of calmness. Remember, worry is connected to the Spleen, and Patchouli has the ability to calm the Shen and strengthen the Spleen. I most often use this oil when there is anxiety accompanied by digestive disturbance, or when there is simply worry and anxiety.

Level of Qi:
Yuan

Fragrance note:
Base

Part of the plant:
Leaves

Temperature:
Slightly warming

Meridian/organ:
Lungs, Stomach, Spleen, Heart

Element:
Earth

Blends well with:
Blood orange, lemongrass, neroli, sweet fennel

Physical actions:
Calms the Shen; relaxes the nervous system; supports digestion

Emotional actions:
Eases anxiety and worry

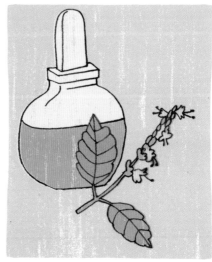

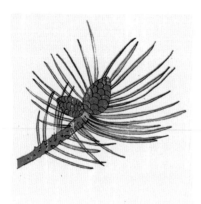

Scots pine (*Pinus sylvestris*)

CLEAN, CLEAR, AND DIRECT

Scots pine essential oil is warming and tonifying, and it has a crisp balsam scent. Scots pine has a long history of being used in cough syrups and cold remedies to assist in expelling phlegm.

Scots pine is connected to the Lungs and Kidneys, and, just like tea tree (see page 74), it can tonify both the Lung Qi and Kidney Qi. Scots pine is often used to expel phlegm from the lungs, tonify the Lungs, and to bring relief to achy muscles. It can be used in a bath with ravensara and tea tree oils to alleviate the muscle aches associated with the common cold. Its tonification properties make it an ideal choice to strengthen the Wei Qi (see page 14) after a common cold or illness.

Scots pine strengthens the Kidney Qi, and it is known to benefit the three cardinal signs of Kidney Qi deficiency: low willpower, low libido, and lower back pain. Scots pine is also beneficial to strengthen the Kidney system when it is deficient due to overwork or stress.

This is a key oil for those who tend to dwell on the past, holding on to regret or guilt. When we tonify the Lung Qi, we are allowing ourselves to take in current life force, which is symbolic of being in the present moment.

Phlegm is a physical blockage that can obstruct breath patterns. However, on an emotional level, those with excess mucus or phlegm may be holding on to negative experiences that lead to low self-confidence. Combining Scots pine with frankincense can break up or transform phlegm to aid in deeper breathing.

Scots pine's warming nature, analgesic properties, and its connection to the Kidney system are all functions that make it a key oil for treating Cold Bi (see page 128). There are many oils that it can be blended with to help alleviate Cold Bi, including vetiver, ginger, sandalwood, *Eucalyptus globulus*, ravensara, tea tree, and sweet marjoram.

Level of Qi:
Ying

Fragrance note:
Middle

Part of the plant:
Needles

Temperature:
Warming

Meridian/organ:
Lung, Kidney

Element:
Metal, Water

Blends well with:
Frankincense, lemongrass, rosemary, tea tree

Physical actions:
Tonifies the Lung Qi and Kidney Qi; eases lower back pain and muscle pain and weakness; increases male libido

Emotional actions:
Helps bring closure; strengthens willpower

CAUTION: Using Scots pine

Scots pine oil is high in alpha-pinene, which means that it oxidizes quickly[3]. To avoid oxidization, the oil should be stored in the refrigerator. If the oil has oxidized, it may cause skin sensitivity.

Sandalwood (*Santalum album*)

CONTEMPLATIVE AND MEDITATIVE

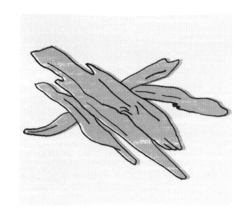

The sandalwood tree (*Santalum album*) is native to India. However, India has placed restrictions on the harvesting of the wood. Today, Australia is the only source of *Santalum album* that has been grown in an ecologically responsible manner. *Santalum spicatum* is also grown in Australia and Indonesia, and its scent and actions are similar to *Santalum album*.

Sandalwood has been used for thousands of years to set the intention, become closer to the divine, prepare for mediation, and to find centeredness within. Its first mention in Indian literature dates back 4,000 years, and sandalwood has been used in Chinese herbal medicine for millennia. Sandalwood is considered to be the choice oil for mediation and contemplation—often it is placed on the Yintang (an acupressure point between the eyebrows, often called the third eye) for this purpose.

The sandalwood tree is a hemiparasitic plant, which means that it attaches its roots to other trees in order to ensure survival. A sandalwood tree can take decades to grow to its full size, just as it takes decades of experience to gain wisdom.

Sandalwood is a natural aphrodisiac for men, and the oil can be blended with clove or cinnamon for this purpose. Sandalwood also has a cooling effect on the skin, and a paste of sandalwood can be used to treat skin irritation.

Level of Qi:
Yuan

Fragrance note:
Base

Part of the plant:
Wood

Temperature:
Cooling

Meridian/organ:
Heart, Kidney

Element:
Fire, Water

Blends well with:
Bergamot, cinnamon, frankincense, geranium, ginger, neroli, patchouli, rose, vetiver

Physical actions:
Calms the mind; nourishes the Heart

Emotional actions:
Promotes meditation, understanding, and acceptance

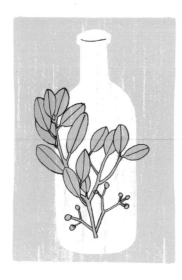

Level of Qi:
Wei-Ying

Fragrance note:
Top-middle

Part of the plant:
Leaves

Temperature:
Cooling

Meridian/organ:
Lung

Element:
Metal

Blends well with:
Eucalyptus globulus,
Eucalyptus radiata,
lemongrass, sweet marjoram

Physical actions:
Tonifies the Lung Qi; eases
muscle aches and pains

Emotional actions:
Eases grief and sadness

Ravensara (*Ravensara aromatica*)

A SYMBOL OF PERSONAL INTEGRITY

Ravensara (also known as clove nutmeg) has a cooling yet spicy scent. This essential oil will go to the Ying level (see page 30), which is associated with the emotions.

Quite often when we are in a state of loss or grief we need assistance in being present to our daily responsibilities. The Lung is the organ most closely associated with breath, and it is also the organ most connected to being present. Lung Qi naturally wants to be proficient and productive, and ravensara can assist in this process. We are more vulnerable to illness when our Lung Qi or Wei Qi (see page 30) is weak. Ravensara will not only strengthen our Lung Qi, but also Release the Exterior (see page 14), and perhaps help us to be more present in the physical world and not to dwell on the past. Ravensara can also be used for the treatment of the common cold and flu, allowing us to proceed with our daily duties.

According to Jeffery Yuen, one of my teachers, ravensara brings relaxation to the erector spinae muscles (a group of muscles attached to the spine). Does this relate to the Lung Qi? Well, the Lungs and the Metal element are both associated with personal integrity (see pages 34–35), and the spine symbolically represents integrity. If a person's spine is aligned then their body is upright and they can take in deep breaths. However, people with a chronic Lung Qi deficiency will often appear to be hunched over, and when someone is in that position they find it difficult to take deep breaths. When the spine is aligned, breathing is regulated and the Kidneys can "grasp" the Lung Qi.

CAUTION: Using ravensara

Ravensara is potentially carcinogenic due to its estragole content, so it is recommended to use the oil at only 1% concentration[4]. Also, because it is high in limonene content, it should be stored in an airtight container in the refrigerator to avoid oxidation.

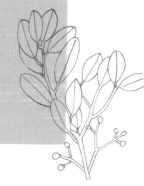

Ginger (*Zingiber officinalis*)

SPICY, MOVING, AND STRENGTHENING

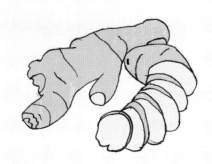

Ginger is a very warm and spicy essential oil. Oil distilled from fresh ginger has a lighter and more fragrant scent than oil distilled from dried ginger, which is generally thicker and has a more inward quality.

We need an adequate amount of warmth and Qi to promote a proper bowel movement. Since ginger is warming, moving, and strengthening, it is commonly used to aid in digestion and peristalsis.

Ginger is most commonly used for digestive disorders that are worse with cold, and for pain that is worse with cold. Therefore, ginger is a suitable choice for disorders that are due to a Spleen and Kidney Qi deficiency.

Ginger tonifies the Spleen Qi and Kidney Qi. The Spleen controls the muscles, so if the Spleen Qi is deficient, then the muscles won't be as strong as they could be. To a greater or lesser extent, strong muscles are linked with willpower. The Kidneys are also associated with willpower and endurance, so you can see the dependent nature of the Spleen Qi on the Kidney Qi.

Damp-Cold Bi (see page 128) is a common ailment that is treated with Chinese medicine. Common symptoms include muscle, joint, or bone pain that is worse with cold. In Western medicine, these symptoms are often diagnosed as arthritis. Ginger is often blended with frankincense, myrrh, sweet marjoram, ravensara, tea tree, clove, or cinnamon to treat Damp-Cold Bi.

Level of Qi:
Ying

Fragrance note:
Middle

Part of the plant:
Roots

Temperature:
Warming

Meridian/organ:
Lung, Spleen, Stomach, Kidney

Element:
Fire, Earth

Blends well with:
Cardamom, patchouli, sandalwood, vetiver

Physical actions:
Eases fatigue, muscle and joint pain that is worse with cold (especially pain in the lower back, hips, and knees); supports digestion; warms the meridians; tonifies Spleen Yang

Emotional actions:
Promotes courage, confidence, endurance, and willpower

CAUTION: Using ginger

Due to ginger's warming nature, this essential oil is contraindicated for children. It should be used with caution when there are signs of Yin deficiency, such as hot flashes (flushes), night sweats, mood swings, and insomnia.

Level of Qi:
Wei, Ying

Fragrance note:
Top, middle

Part of the plant:
Leaf, and sometimes
flowers

Temperature:
Warming

Meridian/organ:
Lung, Spleen, Liver,
Gall Bladder

Element:
Earth, Metal, Wood

Blends well with:
Eucalyptus globulus,
lavender, peppermint,
sweet marjoram

Physical actions:
Eases fatigue, muscle
weakness, and digestive
ailments; prevents the
common cold; raises Yang
Qi; raises and tonifies the
Spleen Qi; raises and
promotes the movement of
Liver Qi; tonifies the Lung Qi

Emotional actions:
Eases irritability and
frustration; boosts low
self-confidence

Rosemary (*Rosmarinus officinalis*)

QI MOVER AND QI ASCENDER

Rosemary is a warming essential oil that is prized for its ability to raise and tonify the Spleen Qi, raise and promote the movement of Liver Qi, and tonify the Lung Qi. When rosemary is used in a blend it is the king—where the energy of rosemary goes, so the other oils follow. Lavender can be used to cool and calm rosemary's raising nature.

Rosemary's ability to Release the Exterior (see page 14), tonify the Lung Qi and Spleen Qi, raise Spleen Yang, and raise Qi is integral when treating many digestive complaints (see Chapter 5).

When Spleen Qi is deficient it descends and does not send pure Qi upward. One of the effects of Spleen Qi deficiency is Dampness (see page 39). Rosemary is key in helping to alleviate symptoms of Dampness, including feelings of heaviness, loose stools, and mental fatigue. Worry often accompanies the physical symptoms of Spleen Qi deficiency. Rosemary can assist us in alleviating worries because it has the ability to raise the Liver Qi.

Rosemary is commonly known as a symbol of remembrance, and recent studies have confirmed that link, showing that rosemary is rich in 1,8 cineole, a compound that can improve focus and concentration. Our intellect and focus is strong when the Spleen is strong.

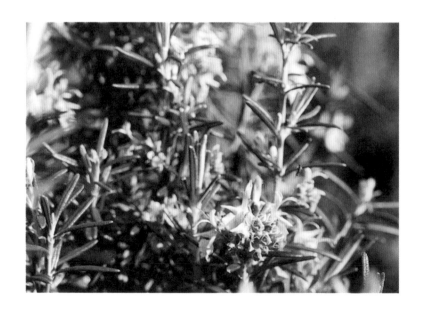

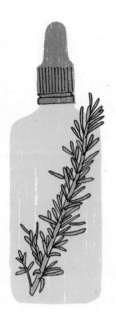

Common Chemotypes of Rosemary

Some essential oils have different chemical compositions (and therefore different therapeutic properties), even though they are obtained from plants that are botanically identical. Such oils are distinguished by chemotype—their most abundant chemical constituent. Camphor, eucalyptol (also known as 1,8 cineole), pinene, and verbenone are all examples of chemotypes.

Essential oils that are named by chemotype include basil, lavender, rosemary, and thyme. For example, Rosemary's common chemotypes include:

- *Rosmarinus officinalis* ct. camfor: It has the highest camphor content, and it is the best rosemary oil to use for muscle aches. It can also be used to stimulate and awaken the mind.
- *Rosmarinus officinalis* ct. cineole: It has the highest 1,8 cineole content, and is commonly used for respiratory ailments.
- *Rosmarinus officinalis* ct. verbenone: It is commonly thought of as the softest rosemary oil, and it has the most pleasant aroma.

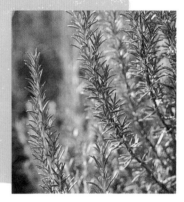

Rosemary also has the ability to raise the Spleen Yang, which is beneficial for developing assertiveness and confidence. Rosemary also strengthens the Spleen, which helps to close our pores to prevent common colds. This function is important because we need strong boundaries to defend ourselves against external pathogenic influences (see page 37) and negative energy from personal relationships.

Rosemary can help to balance our internal terrain. If you look at the way the rosemary plant grows, it generally grows upward and outward, sharing its energetic direction with the world. The essential oil has a similar effect upon the direction of our body's Qi.

CAUTION: Using rosemary

Rosemary oil should not be used close to the face of infants and young children up to the age of five.

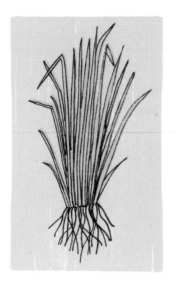

Level of Qi:
Yuan

Fragrance note:
Base

Part of the plant:
Roots

Temperature:
Cooling

Meridian/organ:
Heart, Stomach,
Spleen, Kidney

Element:
Fire, Earth, Water

Blends well with:
Ginger, patchouli,
sandalwood

Physical actions:
Supports the Spleen and
Stomach; calms the mind;
promotes groundedness

Emotional actions:
Eases worry and anxiety

Vetiver (*Vetiveria zizanoides*)

ROOTED, STABLE, AND NOURISHING

Vetiver (also known as the oil of tranquility) is one of the thickest and most viscous of the essential oils. It has a deep-brown amber color that is similar to the color of soil after it has rained. Vetiver oil is distilled from the roots of the plant, and it has an earthy, mysterious, and sensual aroma.

The main organs and meridians that vetiver is associated with are the Spleen, Stomach, and Kidneys. As the oil is a base note, it is also connected to the reproductive system, and to deeper aspects of our being. Vetiver nourishes our Yin and Blood. It is very beneficial for mood swings, the inability to make decisions, and for people who are looking to feel rooted and grounded. Vetiver has a strong affinity to the lower body, especially the lower lumbar region, sacrum (the base of the spine), ankles, and soles of the feet.

Vetiver can promote deep and meaningful relaxation (see page 143 for a simple treatment with vetiver). It is relaxing to the nervous system and the muscular system. It can be blended with lemongrass, frankincense, and sweet marjoram to relax the muscles and sinews.

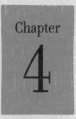

Chapter

4

Essential Oils for the Respiratory System

Aromatherapy is a very effective treatment for the respiratory system. Most of the essential oils associated with the Lung system are made from peels, leaves, and needles. These oils have the ability to Release the Exterior (see page 14) and tonify the Lung Qi, and many of them are also prized for their antibacterial properties.

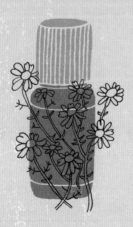

Respiratory Disorders

The main Traditional Chinese Medicine (TCM) diagnoses that we see with the respiratory system are: Wei Qi deficiency, Wind-Heat, Wind-Cold, Lung Qi deficiency, and Phlegm in the Lungs.

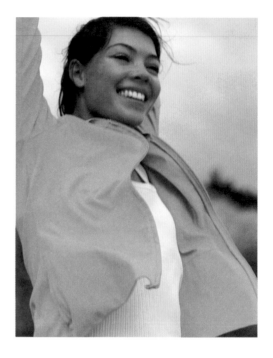

WEI QI DEFICIENCY

Wei Qi (see page 14) is associated with the superficial aspects of the body, and it resides between the skin and the muscles. Wei Qi can be thought of as a wall of defense from external pathogens or anything "negative" from the outside world. When our Wei Qi is strong, we have clear boundaries and adequate energy to perform our daily tasks. When our Wei Qi is deficient, our body is naturally going to be weaker. As you will see later on in this chapter, in order to have strong Wei Qi, and thereby strong Lung Qi, we also need to have a healthy digestive system—or in other words, a vital postnatal Qi (see page 24).

Wind is one of the external factors of illness in Chinese medicine (see page 37), and it is synonymous with change. We need to have adequate Wei Qi in order to move through life's transitions, challenges, and tribulations. If our Wei Qi is weak, we may succumb to common colds, flu, or even pneumonia.

WIND-HEAT AND WIND-COLD

Chinese Medicine classifies the common cold into two types: Wind-Heat and Wind-Cold. The treatment principle for both Wind-Cold and Wind-Heat is the same: Releasing the Exterior. However, the oil combinations are different. Generally speaking, we want to use two cooling oils and one warming oil for Wind-Heat and two warming oils and one cooling oil for Wind-Cold. Such blends should include primarily top note oils to assist in Releasing the Exterior and perhaps one middle note oil to assist in tonifying the Lungs and Wei Qi.

The Common Cold in Chinese Medicine

WIND-COLD	WIND-HEAT
Aversion to cold and wind	Aversion to wind
Chills with no fever	Chills with fever (fever predominant)
Scratchy throat	Sore throat
Runny nose with clear nasal discharge	Yellow nasal discharge
No thirst	Thirst

LUNG QI DEFICIENCY

Common symptoms of Lung Qi deficiency include shortness of breath, spontaneous sweating, frequent common colds, a weak cough, and an aversion to cold. In Chinese medicine, all the organs rely on one another, which means that the Lungs are not solely responsible for their lack of adequate Qi. Lung Qi deficiency is often caused by a Spleen Qi and Kidney Qi deficiency. As a quick reminder, the Lungs are dependent upon the ability of the Spleen to transform postnatal Qi into pure Qi and transport it to the Lungs, and it is the warming function of the Kidneys that gives the Spleen the ability to function properly. Therefore, you will notice that the oils that strengthen Lung Qi, such as tea tree and rosemary, are also associated with the Kidney.

PHLEGM IN THE LUNGS

Congestion can develop in the lungs when there is a Lung Qi deficiency. This is for two reasons. First, when Spleen Qi is weak it leads to Dampness (see page 39)—according to Chinese medicine the Spleen produces Dampness, which is stored in the Lungs. Second, when Lung Qi is weak it does not have the power to circulate the Qi in the chest, and so phlegm accumulates.

Many of the same oils that are used to strengthen the Lungs and Release the Exterior are also used to expel phlegm. Phlegm is expelled through coughing, so a cough may become worse for a couple of days.

Blends to Aid the Respiratory System

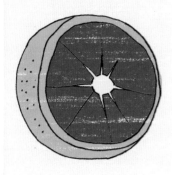

USING BLOOD ORANGE TO RELIEVE WIND-HEAT BY RELEASING THE EXTERIOR

You will need
5-ml blending bottle
Jojoba oil
6 drops blood orange oil

1 Fill the bottle with 1 teaspoon (5 ml) jojoba oil, then add the blood orange oil and shake for a few moments.
2 Put two or three drops of the oil blend on the Large Intestine 1 point (**LI 1**). Using your thumb or index finger, gently massage 27 small circles over the point.
3 Put two or three drops of the oil blend on the Lung 11 point (**LU 11**). Using your thumb or index finger, gently massage 27 small circles over the point.

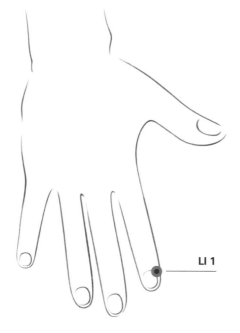

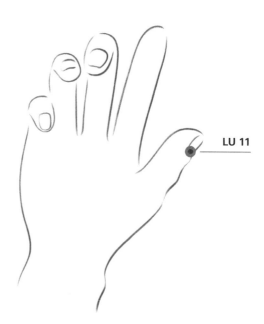

LU 11

LI 1

A BLEND TO SUPPORT RESPIRATION

This exercise should be done three times per day. It will tonify the Lung Qi and Kidney Qi, open up the chest, and increase the depth of breathing.

You will need

10-ml blending bottle

Jojoba oil

4 drops tea tree oil

2 drops frankincense oil

1 drop bergamot oil

1 Fill the bottle with 2 teaspoons (10 ml) jojoba oil, then add the tea tree, frankincense, and bergamot oils and shake for a few moments.
2 Use the palm inhalation technique (see page 49) to inhale one drop of the oil blend.
3 Put one drop of the oil blend on the Lung 9 point (**LU 9**). Using your thumb or index finger, gently massage 9 to 27 small circles over the point. This will tonify the Lung Qi.
4 Put one drop of the oil blend on your thumb or index finger and then place the oil on the Ren 17 point (**RN 17**). Gently massage 9 to 27 small circles over the point. This will open up the chest.
5 Put one drop of the oil blend on your thumb or index finger and then place the oil on the Kidney 7 point (**KD 7**). Gently massage 9 to 27 small circles over the point. This will tonify the Lung Qi and help with inner will.
6 Use the palm inhalation technique to inhale one drop of the oil blend.

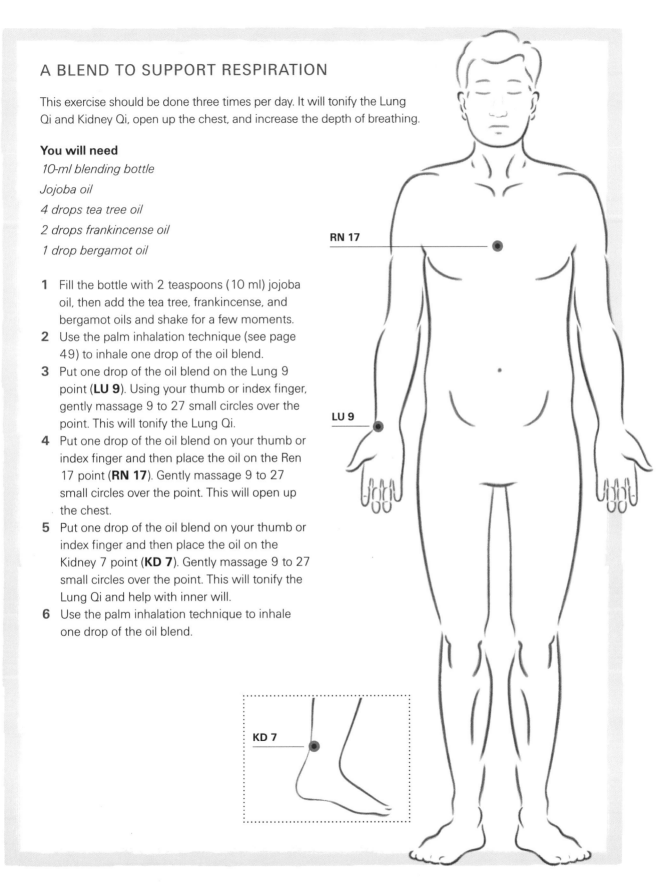

RN 17

LU 9

KD 7

USING PEPPERMINT FOR AN ACUTE STIFF NECK

You will need

5-ml blending bottle

Jojoba oil

8 to 10 drops peppermint oil

Warm moist compress (see page 52)

Towel

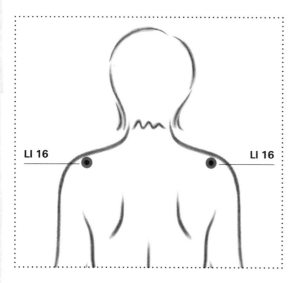

1 Fill the bottle with 1 teaspoon (5 ml) jojoba oil, then add the peppermint oil and shake for a few moments.

2 Put ten drops of the oil blend in the palm of your hand. Massage the back of your neck and down the trapezius muscles (the upper and back part of the neck and shoulders) to the Large Intestine 16 point (**LI 16**) on your right shoulder. Repeat this 27 times.

3 Adding a few more drops of the peppermint blend to the palm of your hand if necessary, massage the back of your neck and down the trapezius muscles to the Large Intestine 16 point (**LI 16**) on your left shoulder. Repeat this 27 times.

4 Apply a warm moist compress to the painful area of your neck, cover it with a dry towel, and hold it in place until the compress cools.

USING PEPPERMINT FOR SINUS CONGESTION

Blend 1

You will need

Large bowl

2 to 4 drops peppermint oil

Towel

1 Fill a bowl with boiling water. Let the water cool for a few minutes, then add two drops of peppermint oil (start with just two drops and then add more if necessary) and mix well to allow the vapors to rise into the air.

2 Place a towel over your head and then carefully lower your face over the bowl until your face is 6 to 8 inches (15 to 20 cm) above the water. Close your eyes and inhale slowly through your nose for a few seconds, then lift your head up and exhale.

3 Repeat the inhalation and exhalation process three to five times.

Blend 2

You will need

2 drops peppermint oil

2 drops Eucalyptus radiata *oil*

1 Turn on the shower and let the hot water run for a minute.
2 Put the drops of peppermint and eucalyptus oils on the floor of the shower.
3 Step into the shower and begin to feel better.

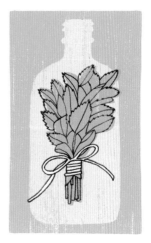

Blend 3

You will need

5-ml blending bottle

Jojoba oil

8 to 10 drops peppermint oil

1 Fill the bottle with 1 teaspoon (5 ml) jojoba oil, then add the peppermint oil and shake for a few moments.
2 Put one drop of the oil blend on each of your index fingers and then place the oil on the Large Intestine 20 points (**LI 20**) on either side of your face, taking slow deep breaths.
3 Put two drops of the oil blend on each of your index fingers and then place the oil on the Gall Bladder 20 points (**GB 20**) on either side of your head. Gently massage the oil over the points with a circular motion.

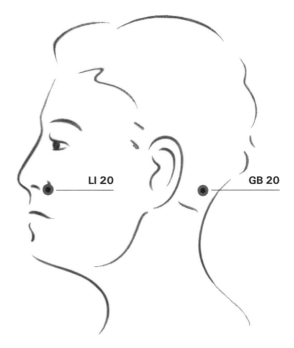

AN EXPECTORANT TO EXPEL YELLOW PHLEGM

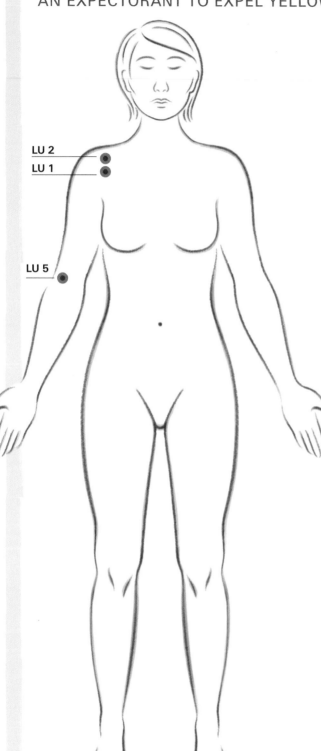

LU 2
LU 1
LU 5

You will need

5-ml blending bottle

Jojoba oil

3 drops Eucalyptus radiata *oil*

1 drop tea tree oil

1 drop basil linalool oil

Warm moist compress (see page 52)

Towel

1 Fill the bottle with 1 teaspoon (5 ml) jojoba oil, then add the eucalyptus, tea tree, and basil oils and shake for a few moments.

2 Put three drops of the oil blend on the Lung 5 point (**LU 5**). Using your thumb or index finger, gently massage nine small circles over the point.

3 Put three drops of the oil blend on your thumb or index finger and then place the oil on the Lung 1 point (**LU 1**). Gently massage the oil over the point with a circular motion.

4 Put three drops of the oil blend on your thumb or index finger and then place the oil on the Lung 2 point (**LU 2**). Gently massage the oil over the point with a circular motion.

5 With a loose fist, gently tap the Lung 1 and Lung 2 points (**LU 1** and **LU 2**) for 30 seconds.

6 Lie down on your back and take a few deep breaths. Place a warm moist compress on your upper chest and cover it with a dry towel. With a loose fist, gently tap on your chest for 1 to 2 minutes. (If you have a partner to help you, this step should also be repeated on your upper back.)

A SHOWER SCRUB FOR THE COMMON COLD

This is a body scrub that you can use in the shower when you feel as if you are coming down with a cold.

You will need

1 to 2 drops Eucalyptus radiata *oil*

1 teaspoon sea salt

Small container

2 teaspoons jojoba oil

1 Place the eucalyptus oil and sea salt in a small container. Cover with jojoba oil.
2 Step into a hot shower. Gently massage one-third of the scrub in your hands and then vigorously massage the scrub up and down your inner arm (the palm side) and all the way up to the back of your neck nine times.
3 Repeat the massage on the opposite arm.

A BATH TO RELIEVE COLDS AND MUSCLE ACHES

You will need

2 teapoons (10 ml) liquid Castile soap (or you can use vegetable or jojoba oil)

3 drops ravensara oil (tonifies the Lung Qi, relaxes muscles, and alleviates pain)

1 drop tea tree oil (tonifies the Lung Qi, relaxes muscles, and alleviates pain)

1 drop Eucalyptus radiata *oil (Releases the Exterior)*

1 drop sweet marjoram oil (Releases the Exterior and relaxes muscles)

Small bowl

1 Mix together the soap and essential oils in a small bowl.
2 Fill a bathtub with hot water, then add the soap mixture and swirl to mix well.
3 Get into the bath and soak in the water for about 20 minutes.

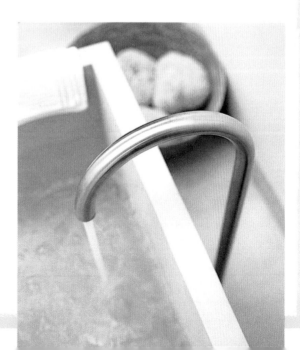

A BLEND TO IMPROVE LUNG VITALITY

This treatment with tonify the Lung Qi.

You will need

5-ml blending bottle

Jojoba oil

2 drops Eucalyptus radiata *oil*

1 drop ravensara oil

1 drop basil linalool oil

1 Fill the bottle with 1 teaspoon (5 ml) jojoba oil, then add the eucalyptus, ravensara, and basil oils and shake for a few moments.
2 Put one drop of the oil blend on your thumb or index finger and then place the oil on the Ren 17 point (**RN 17**). Gently massage the oil over the point with a circular motion. Ren 17 is one of the influential points of Qi—a point that has a strong effect on a broad area or function of the body.
3 Put one drop of the oil blend on the Lung 9 point (**LU 9**). Using your thumb or index finger, gently massage the oil over the point with a circular motion. This will tonify the Lung Qi.
4 Put one drop of the oil blend on your thumb or index finger and then place the oil on the Kidney 7 point (**KD 7**). Gently massage the oil over the point with a circular motion. This will help to strengthen your will.

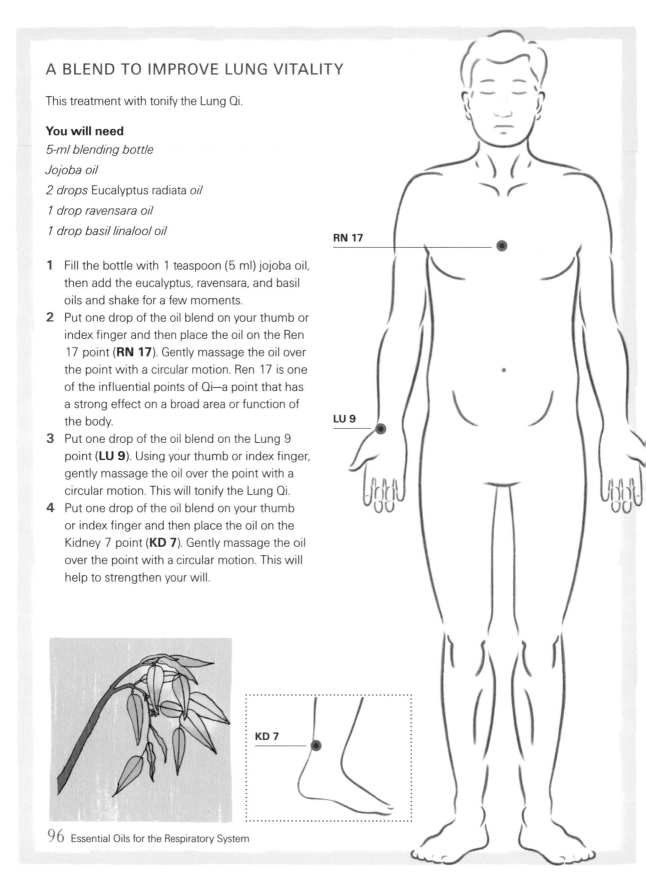

A SIMPLE LUNG STRENGTHENER

This may aid the symptoms of a Qi deficiency, such as a low voice, dislike of speaking, or fatigue. It is also good for someone who experiences frequent common colds.

You will need

5-ml blending bottle

Jojoba oil

2 drops tea tree oil

1 drop Scots pine oil

1 drop frankincense oil

1 Fill the bottle with 1 teaspoon (5 ml) jojoba oil, then add the tea tree, Scots pine, and frankincense oils and shake for a few moments.

2 Put one drop of the oil blend on your thumb or index finger and then place the oil on the Ren 17 point (**RN 17**)—one of the influential points of Qi. Gently massage three to nine small circles over the point.

3 Put one drop of the oil blend on the Lung 9 point (**LU 9**). Gently massage small circles over the point, and then massage up and down the Lung meridian three to nine times. This will tonify the Lung Qi.

4 Put one drop of the oil blend on your thumb or index finger and then place the oil on the Kidney 7 point (**KD 7**). Gently massage nine small circles over the point. This will help to strengthen your will.

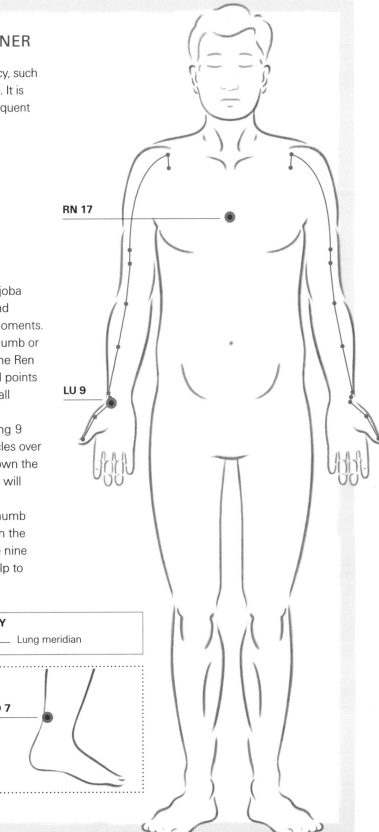

RN 17

LU 9

KEY

Lung meridian

KD 7

A BLEND FOR THE SYMPTOMS OF WIND-COLD

You will need

5-ml blending bottle

Jojoba oil

2 drops peppermint oil

2 drops basil linalool oil

1 drop Eucalyptus radiata *oil*

1 drop Eucalyptus globulus *oil*

1 Fill the bottle with 1 teaspoon (5 ml) jojoba oil, then add the peppermint, basil, and eucalyptus oils and shake for a few moments.

2 Put one drop of the oil blend on the Lung 7 point (**LU 7**). Using your thumb or index finger, gently massage nine small circles over the point, then massage all the way up and down the Lung meridian nine times, adding more jojoba oil if necessary. This will release Wind-Cold and disperse Cold.

3 Put one drop of the oil blend on your thumb or index finger and then place the oil on the Large Intestine 20 point (**LI 20**). Gently massage nine small circles over the point. This will open the nasal passages.

4 Put one drop of the oil blend on your thumb or index finger and then place the oil on the Urinary Bladder 60 point (**UB 60**). Gently massage nine small circles over the point. This will Release the Exterior.

5 Put one drop of the oil blend on your thumb or index finger and then place the oil on the Urinary Bladder 13 point (**UB 13**)—this is the back shu point (see box right) of the Lung. Gently massage nine small circles over the point.

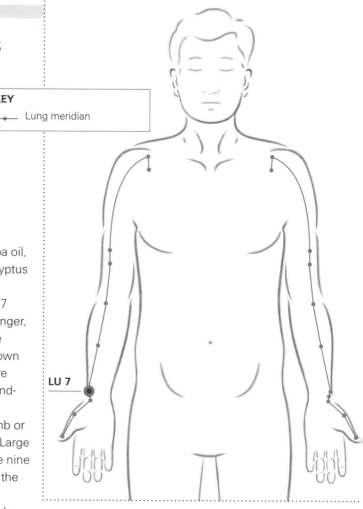

KEY	
•——	Lung meridian

LU 7

Back Shu Points

The back shu points are located on the Urinary Bladder meridian. Each shu point is infused with the energy of a specific organ, and each point is in direct communication with its organ. The back shu points are most often used to regulate and tonify the organs.

If you find it difficult to reach the back shu points, you may find it helpful to ask a friend or partner to apply the oil to those points.

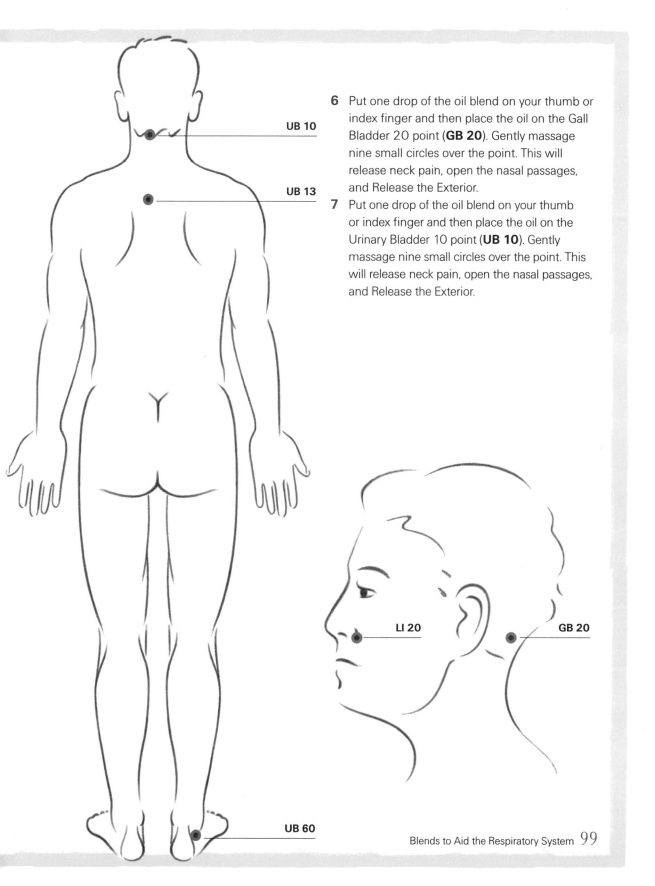

UB 10

UB 13

UB 60

6   Put one drop of the oil blend on your thumb or index finger and then place the oil on the Gall Bladder 20 point (**GB 20**). Gently massage nine small circles over the point. This will release neck pain, open the nasal passages, and Release the Exterior.

7   Put one drop of the oil blend on your thumb or index finger and then place the oil on the Urinary Bladder 10 point (**UB 10**). Gently massage nine small circles over the point. This will release neck pain, open the nasal passages, and Release the Exterior.

LI 20

GB 20

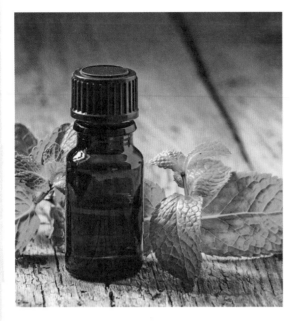

A BLEND FOR CONGESTION AND NECK PAIN

This treatment can be used for congestion and the neck pain caused by Wind-Cold (see page 88).

You will need

5-ml blending bottle
Jojoba oil
2 drops basil linalool oil
2 drops peppermint oil

1 Fill the bottle with 1 teaspoon (5 ml) jojoba oil, then add the basil and peppermint oils and shake for a few moments.
2 Use the palm inhalation technique (see page 49) to inhale five drops of the oil blend.
3 Using the palm of your hand, gently massage the back of your neck with a circular motion, paying particular attention to any tender areas.
4 If you are suffering from congestion, put one drop of the oil blend on each of your index fingers and then gently press them into the Large Intestine 20 points (**LI 20**) on either side of your face. Gently massage 9 to 27 small circles over the points.

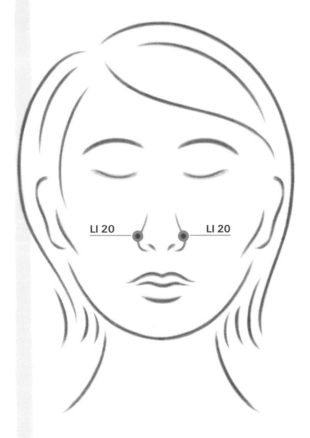

LI 20   LI 20

A BLEND TO RELIEVE LUNG CONGESTION

This treatment can be used for congestion in the lungs due to Wind-Cold (see page 88).

You will need

5-ml blending bottle

Jojoba oil

2 drops Eucalyptus globulus *oil (Releases the Exterior, expels phlegm, and opens the chest)*

2 drops Eucalyptus radiata *oil (Releases the Exterior, expels phlegm, and opens the chest)*

2 drops basil linalool oil (Releases the Exterior)

Warm moist compress (see page 52)

Towel

1 Fill the bottle with 1 teaspoon (5 ml) jojoba oil, then add the eucalyptus and basil oils and shake for a few moments.
2 Put two drops of the oil blend on the Large Intestine 4 point (**LI 4**). Using your thumb or index finger, gently massage nine circles over the point.
3 Put four drops of the oil blend on your thumb or index finger. Using circular motions, massage up and down the Lung and Large Intestine meridians nine times.
4 Put two drops of the oil blend on your thumb or index finger and place the oil on the Lung 1 or Lung 2 point (**LU 1** or **LU 2**), whichever is most tender. Gently massage three to five circles over the point.
5 Lie down on your back. Place a warm moist compress on your chest, cover it with a dry towel, and leave it in place until the compress cools.

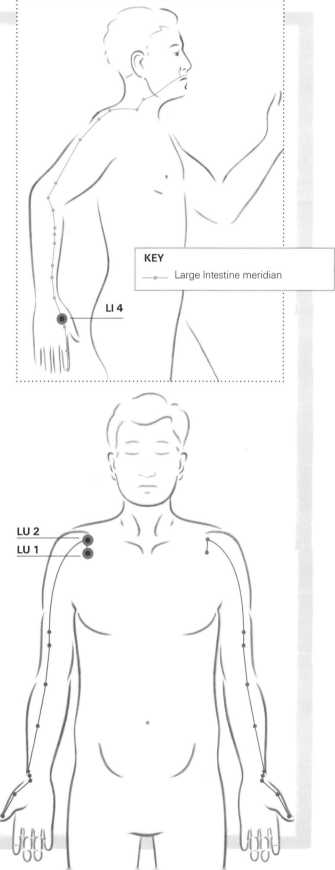

KEY

⊸•⊸ Large Intestine meridian

LI 4

LU 2
LU 1

KEY

⊸•⊸ Lung meridian

A BLEND TO RELIEVE NECK AND UPPER BODY PAIN

This treatment can be used for the neck and upper body pain caused by Wind-Cold (see page 88).

You will need

5-ml blending bottle

Jojoba oil

2 drops Eucalyptus globulus *oil*

2 drops basil linalool oil

2 drops peppermint oil

Warm moist compress (see page 52)

Towel

1 Fill the bottle with 1 teaspoon (5 ml) jojoba oil, then add the eucalyptus, basil, and peppermint oils and shake for a few moments.
2 Put two drops of the oil blend on the Large Intestine 4 point (**LI 4**). Using your thumb or index finger, gently massage nine small circles over the point.
3 Put four drops of the oil blend on your thumb or index finger. Using circular motions, massage up and down the Lung and Large Intestine meridians nine times.
4 Put six drops of the oil blend in the palms of your hand and then gently massage any sore areas.
5 Place a warm moist compress on any tender areas, cover with a dry towel, and hold it in place until the compress cools. You can repeat this step up to three times, if liked.

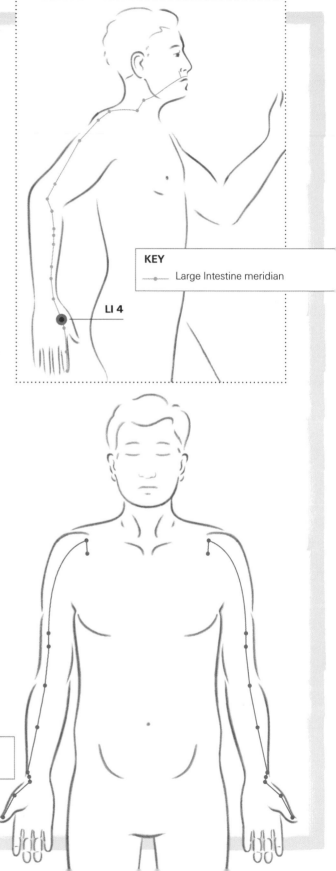

KEY
— Large Intestine meridian

LI 4

KEY
— Lung meridian

A BLEND TO PREVENT THE SYMPTOMS OF THE COMMON COLD AND STRENGTHEN BOUNDARIES

This treatment will prevent the symptoms of Wind-Cold (see page 88), tonify the Lung Qi, and Strengthen Wei Qi (see page 14).

You will need

5-ml blending bottle

Jojoba oil

2 drops rosemary oil (tonifies the Lung Qi and strengthens Wei Qi)

1 drop ravensara oil (tonfies the Lung Qi)

1 drop tea tree oil (tonifies the Lung Qi)

1 drop lemon oil (supports the actions of the other oils)

1 Fill the bottle with 1 teaspoon (5 ml) jojoba oil, then add the rosemary, ravensara, tea tree, and lemon oils and shake for a few moments.

2 Put one drop of the oil blend on the Lung 9 point (**LU 9**). Using your thumb or index finger, gently massage nine small circles over the point, then massage all the way up and down the Lung meridian (see opposite) nine times, adding more jojoba oil if necessary.

3 Put one drop of the oil blend on your thumb or index finger and then place the oil on the Kidney 7 point (**KD 7**). Gently massage nine small circles over the point.

4 Put one drop of the oil blend on your thumb or index finger and then place the oil on the Ren 17 point (**RN 17**). Gently massage nine small circles over the point.

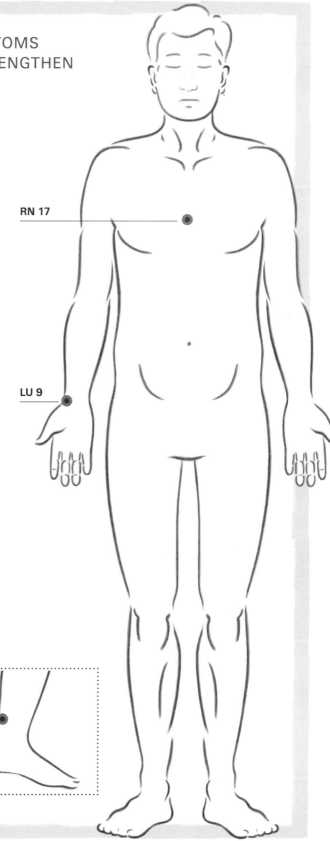

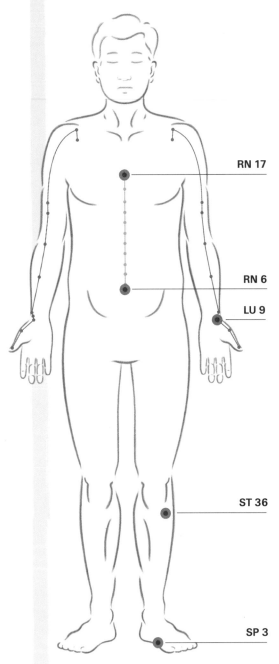

A BLEND TO SUPPORT RESPIRATION AND DIGESTION

This treatment will tonify the Lung and Spleen Qi.

You will need

5-ml blending bottle

Jojoba oil

2 drops rosemary oil (tonifies the Lung Qi and strengthens the Spleen)

2 drops lemongrass oil (revives the Spleen and assists rosemary in raising Spleen Qi)

1 drop sweet fennel oil (tonifies the Spleen and Kidney Qi)

1 drop lemon oil (supports the actions of the other oils)

Warm moist compress (see page 52)

Towel

RN 17

RN 6

LU 9

ST 36

SP 3

1 Fill the bottle with 1 teaspoon (5 ml) jojoba oil, then add the rosemary, lemongrass, sweet fennel, and lemon oils and shake for a few moments.

2 Put one drop of the oil blend on the Lung 9 point (**LU 9**). Using your thumb or index finger, gently massage the oil over the point in a circular motion, then massage up and down the Lung meridian nine times, if liked (massaging the meridian is optional).

3 Put three drops of the oil blend on your thumb or index finger and then place the oil on the Spleen 3 point (**SP 3**). Gently massage nine small circles over the point.

4 Put three drops of the oil blend on your thumb or index finger and then place the oil on the Stomach 36 point (**ST 36**). Gently massage 9 to 27 small circles over the point.

5 Put three drops of the oil blend on your thumb or index finger and then place the oil on the Ren 6 point (**RN 6**). Gently massage 9 to 27 small circles over the point, then stroke upward along the Ren meridian to the Ren 17 point (**RN 17**).

6 Put four drops of the oil blend in the palms of your hand and then gently massage your abdomen.

7 Lie down on your back. Place a warm moist compress on your abdomen, cover it with a dry towel, and leave it in place until the compress cools.

KEY

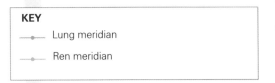

Lung meridian

Ren meridian

Essential Oils to Aid Digestion

A diet rich in nutrients is the key to a life of vitality and health. Without healthy food and proper digestion, our bodies are likely to become vulnerable to illness.

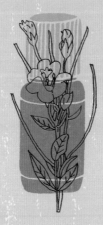

The Digestive System

The Spleen and the Stomach—or the Earth Element—are both associated with digestion. These two organs transform and transport postnatal Qi (see page 24) into internal nourishment and Qi. This transformative process is supported by the warming function of the Kidneys (Kidney Fire).

Digestion begins in the mouth with the chewing of food and the secretion of digestive enzymes—in Traditional Chinese Medicine (TCM), the Spleen is said to open into the mouth. The teeth, which are responsible for proper chewing and the breakdown of food in the mouth, are associated with Jing (see page 23) and bone formation, and they stem from the Kidney Qi.

Many of the oils used for digestion are associated with either the Kidneys or Spleen. Patchouli, rosemary, cardamom, and lemongrass are all associated with the Spleen, while ginger and Scots pine are associated with both the Spleen and Kidneys. All these oils are considered to be warming.

Symptoms of the Liver overacting on the Spleen (see page 109) require oils associated with the Liver, such as lavender, peppermint, and Roman chamomile.

In Chinese Medicine, the Spleen and the Stomach are associated with digestion.

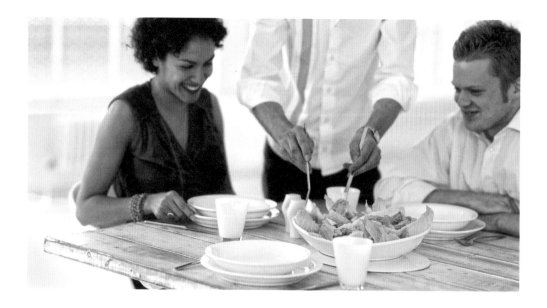

Digestive Disorders

Digestive disturbances can be caused by both physical and emotional factors, and most often these factors cannot be separated. For example, people who are going through difficult changes and experiencing anxiety or depression often try to satiate themselves with food.

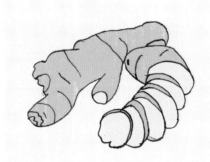

Ginger

Eating sugary foods and candies is one of the quickest ways for people to feel satisfied, as if they've actually accomplished something, but when their blood sugar level eventually crashes, they feel numb. We have all experienced that feeling of being "stuffed" to the point that it has made us feel lazy after overindulging. We only have a certain amount of Qi, and at times like this our Qi is consumed with trying to digest the food we've eaten, leaving us with little energy for anything else.

Food Classification

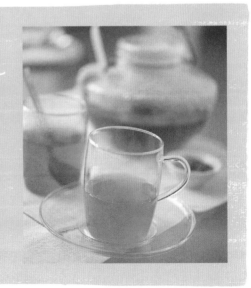

In TCM, foods are classified as Cool, Cold, Warm, Hot, or Neutral. These classifications may refer to the actual temperature of the food, or to the effects that the food has on the body. Cool and Cold foods have a cooling effect on the body, while Warm and Hot foods have a warming effect.

SPLEEN QI DEFICIENCY

The Chinese medicine diagnosis of Spleen Qi deficiency is one of the most commonly seen presentations. Within Chinese medicine theory, the Spleen works in tandem with the Stomach to extract usable nutrients from food and use them to create Qi and Blood. It is at this stage in the digestive process that the body also starts to separate the clear and the turbid, sending waste for evacuation while preserving the usable constituents. This partnership of the Spleen and Stomach is one of the cornerstones of the body microcosm. The health of this relationship fosters or depletes our energy stores and has a big impact on our emotional stability.

The Spleen also governs the growth and health of muscle tissue. Working out and strengthening the muscles can support the Spleen-Stomach, but excessive lifting and labor may damage it.

Improper foods, overthinking (any type of work that requires mental concentration), and physical overwork can all damage the function of the Spleen-Stomach partnership. Cold temperatures and Cold foods can also damage the Spleen-Stomach. Cold foods such as salads, fruit, green drinks, and juices can impair the digestive function when eaten beyond moderation or without balance. Warm foods, such as soups, cooked vegetables, grains, and lean meats, are much more easy to digest. It's best to eat foods that are in season and grown in your local geographic area. Those who live in cold climates would do well to avoid tropical fruits, while those who live below the equator can eat more of these kinds of food.

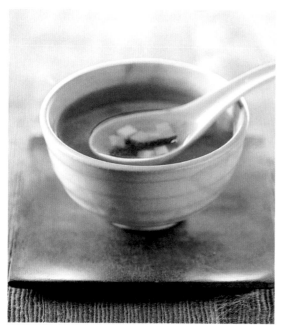

When the Spleen-Stomach becomes damaged, the effects can be seen in the digestive function, energy levels, and emotions. The cardinal sign of Spleen Qi deficiency is abdominal bloating. Changes in bowel movements, such as loose stools, sluggish digestion, alternating constipation and diarrhea, belching, and gas are all common manifestations.

Damage to the Spleen-Stomach affects emotional rootedness. People

It is much easier to digest warm foods, such as soup.

who suffer from this condition often become engaged in worry, anxiety, and obsessive thinking. These emotional changes are the result of the decreased production of Blood from food. Healthy Blood gives us a settled and stable emotional landscape, and the lack of it makes us feel unfocused and nervous.

Many people with Spleen Qi deficiency complain of fatigue, which is caused by the decreased production of Qi. The hallmark description of this type of fatigue is "sinking:" limbs feel tired, heavy, and difficult to move; we feel closer to the floor; and it seems like a chore to keep ourselves upright. In its advanced stages, this type of Spleen Qi deficiency can lead to prolapse, such as hemorrhoids or pelvic floor weakness.

LIVER OVERACTING ON THE SPLEEN

A healthy Spleen has an upward direction: it helps to pull nutrition from our food and sends it upward, and it helps us to build muscle so that we can remain upright. A taxed Spleen has a downward direction, which can be seen with issues of diarrhea and "sinking" fatigue. When the Spleen is damaged, it creates a vacuum for another organ system—the Liver—to fill.

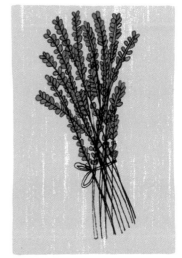

Lavender is used in a blend to ease the Liver overacting on the Spleen (see page 115).

One of the Liver's functions is to maintain the smooth flow of Qi throughout the body. This continuous flow brings nutrition to every cell and organ. The healthy flow of the Liver is omni-directional. Wherever stagnation occurs in this process, illness can arise. For example, when the opposing energy of the Spleen is weak, the Liver asserts itself and takes control.

Wood is the element of the Liver, signified by a young sapling. Rather than an aging oak, this young sapling still has enormous flexibility. It bends easily in the wind but does not snap. The movement of the Liver Qi impacts our emotional processing in the same way. We are meant to experience all emotions (even negative ones such as anger and grief), but only as the wind through the trees—passing through and not retained. When the flow of Liver Qi is impaired, our emotions also become stuck, and we become more prone to outbursts of anger or irritability.

On top of the base symptoms of Spleen Qi deficiency, we may start to see the more aggressive symptoms of Liver Qi stagnation, such as irritability, anger, sighing, upper-right abdominal pain, and tension across the middle of the body. If the Liver is overacting on the Stomach aspect of the Spleen-Stomach partnership, we see acid reflux, nausea, and stomach pain. If the Liver is impacting the Spleen function more, we see diarrhea, often accompanied by cramping.

FOOD STAGNATION

If you've ever overindulged during a celebratory meal, then you've likely experienced food stagnation afterward. The symptoms include indigestion, bloating, belching, and nausea, and it has a temporary effect on the stools too. Most of us, if this is our only indiscretion, will feel back to normal within a day or so. However, food stagnation can become advanced and chronic if we routinely overeat or eat in an imbalanced manner.

Raw and Cold foods (see page 107) can impair the Spleen-Stomach's ability to process foods. The result of that impairment is a buildup of mucus, termed Dampness in Chinese medicine theory (see page 39). This mucus barrier can further impede the proper absorption of nutrients in the gut. The body will also seek to expel this Dampness: stools can become soft or slow moving; allergies can become active, creating a lot of nasal dripping and runny eyes; and skin conditions such as acne may flare. Dampness increases the fatigue experienced with Spleen Qi deficiency.

When this scenario is combined with drinking alcohol or eating spicy or greasy foods, Heat is injected into the situation. In such instances, fluids become more stagnant, and the Dampness congeals further in stickier Phlegm. Soft stools start to move toward chronic constipation. The body's efforts at expelling the Dampness become chronic health conditions, and the more advanced this mucus formation becomes, the more aggressive and long-term the process of resolution will be.

Damp and Phlegm have a strong impact on our mental focus. All our senses tend to become more dulled, but our mental sharpness suffers the most. This can lead to feelings of disengagement and apathy.

Treatments for food stagnation always include changes to diet and addressing the person's relationship with food.

KIDNEY AND SPLEEN YANG DEFICIENCY

The Spleen is one of the primary players in the process of healthy digestion, but it needs direct energy from the Kidneys to complete its digestive duties. The Kidney system is often described as the furnace that fuels the entire body: it is the seat of Yang energy, which is warming and active in nature.

Feeling cold, sometimes described as being "cold to the bones," is often an indicator of a Kidney Yang deficiency (a severe Qi deficiency). Covering up with more clothing will not make this type of cold feel better because it is caused by an internal lack of Yang Qi (see page 30).

The Kidneys are associated with bone health, so pain and weakness of the lower back and knees are often experienced when this system is weakened. The Kidneys also have a relationship with the Urinary Bladder, and a Kidney Qi deficiency can reflect urinary symptoms such as incontinence.

While all of us will naturally lose some Kidney Qi as we grow older, a Kidney Qi deficiency can occur at any age. Often the culprit is some form of a "sex, drugs, and rock 'n' roll" lifestyle. Legal and illegal recreational substances all tax the Kidneys, more so when their use is chronic or extreme.

Sexual function and reproduction also use Kidney Qi (see page 25). Excessive sexual practices and giving birth to lots of children can both impair the function of the Kidney system. Chronic overwork and immersion in stressful environments take their toll in exactly the same manner. For example, veterans returning from war, high-powered executives, and long-term medical carers can all experience symptoms based on depleted Kidney Yang.

When the Kidney Yang is weak, what it gives to the Spleen is diminished as well. This often results in diarrhea that usually occurs right after waking, termed "cock's crow diarrhea." Urine can be voluminous with a pale or clear color. Often eliminations will have little or no smell, a sign of Cold and the absence of warming Yang. The prevailing complaint will be Cold, no matter the environment or season. This pervasive Cold will create aching and stiffness throughout the body. Over time, the impact of impaired nutritional absorption can be seen in pallor, poor skin and hair quality, hearing issues, sexual dysfunction, and premature aging. In such cases, both the Kidney and the Spleen need to be supplemented in order to return the organs to their previous balance, enabling them to create the important building blocks for health.

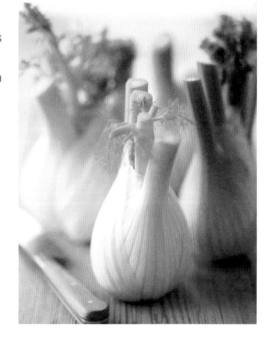

Sweet fennel oil warms the center, strengthens the Kidneys, and stimulates digestion.

Change the Way You Eat

While aromatherapy can enhance digestion and bring relief to many common complaints, holistic healing and holistic aromatherapy also rely on the individual to make positive lifestyle changes.

There are many things that you can do to stimulate proper digestion. One of the most beneficial things to do is to chew your food properly. Chewing food slowly, and up to 50 times per mouthful, makes food easier to digest.

Be mindful about your digestion: think about the time, effort, and labor that go into producing the food you eat. Chewing food slowly is a good way to respect the labor of the people who have helped to bring a meal to your plate.

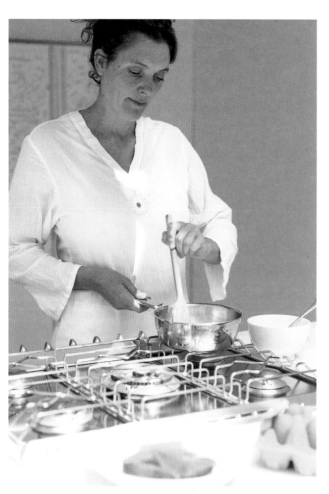

EAT COOKED FOOD

The Spleen thrives on warmth. By warming the Spleen, we are essentially warming the digestive system. In order to maintain a sense of warmth and nourishment, the food that we eat should primarily be composed of foods that are cooked. Too many raw and cold foods will damage the Spleen, inhibiting digestion and Blood formation. Chinese medicine cites this as the reason why many vegans and vegetarians have deficient Blood. Essential oils that benefit digestion, tonify the Spleen, and are warming to the Middle Jiao (see opposite) are important for vegans and vegetarians.

The Three Jiaos

- The Upper Jiao: The Upper Jiao is likened to a canopy. In the same way that a forest canopy forms a highway for the dispersal of water and nutrients, so does the Upper Jiao manage the waterways of the body and the distribution of the Wei Qi (see page 14).
- The Middle Jiao: The job of the Middle Jiao is described as "rotting and ripening." This is the process of the Spleen and Stomach breaking down foods, gathering beneficial nutrients, and sending the remainder to be processed as waste.
- The Lower Jiao: The Lower Jiao is referred to as the "drainage ditch." This Jiao manages the final processing and elimination of solid and fluid waste via the Small and Large Intestines, Kidneys, and Urinary Bladder.

SET YOUR INTENTION

When my clients are looking to make changes in their lives, I often advise them to inhale one essential oil three times a day, and to do this with the intention of making that change. The repetition of using the oil three times per day helps you to actualize intentions and form positive habits.

For digestive disorders, think about using oils that are beneficial for the digestive system, such as fennel, ginger, and cardamom. If your purpose is to stimulate digestion, use Roman chamomile, which comes from a flower and helps harmonize the Spleen. Another oil that can be used for this purpose is neroli. As far as I am aware, neroli is the only floral oil that has the ability to tonify the Spleen Qi and nourish the Blood.

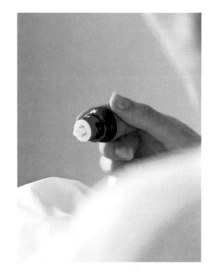

Opposite: Try to eat cooked food to warm the Spleen.

Right: Creating a routine of inhaling one essential oil three times a day helps you set, remember, and follow through with your intention.

Blends to Aid Digestion

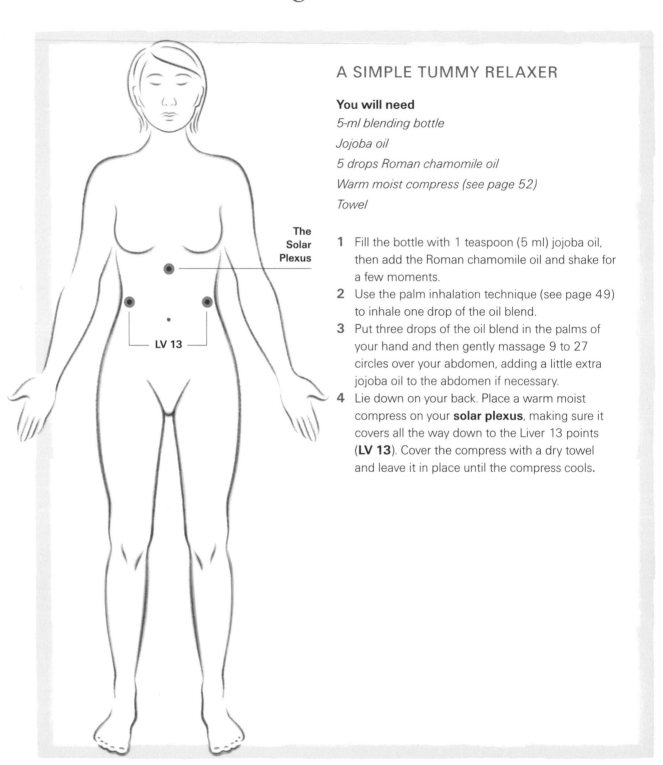

The Solar Plexus

LV 13

A SIMPLE TUMMY RELAXER

You will need
5-ml blending bottle
Jojoba oil
5 drops Roman chamomile oil
Warm moist compress (see page 52)
Towel

1 Fill the bottle with 1 teaspoon (5 ml) jojoba oil, then add the Roman chamomile oil and shake for a few moments.
2 Use the palm inhalation technique (see page 49) to inhale one drop of the oil blend.
3 Put three drops of the oil blend in the palms of your hand and then gently massage 9 to 27 circles over your abdomen, adding a little extra jojoba oil to the abdomen if necessary.
4 Lie down on your back. Place a warm moist compress on your **solar plexus**, making sure it covers all the way down to the Liver 13 points (**LV 13**). Cover the compress with a dry towel and leave it in place until the compress cools.

A BLEND FOR LIVER OVERACTING ON THE SPLEEN

This treatment will have positive effects on indigestion, nausea, abdominal bloating, diarrhea, acid reflux, irritability, and frustration.

You will need

5-ml blending bottle

Jojoba oil

3 drops Roman chamomile oil

2 drops lavender oil

1 drop lemongrass oil

Warm moist compress (see page 52)

Towel

1 Fill the bottle with 1 teaspoon (5 ml) jojoba oil, then add the Roman chamomile, lavender, and lemongrass oils and shake for a few moments.

2 Use the palm inhalation technique (see page 49) to inhale one drop of the oil blend.

3 Put two drops of the oil blend on your thumb or index finder and then place the oil on the Ren 12 point (**RN 12**). Using the palm of your hand, massage 18 circles over the point, adding a little extra jojoba oil if needed. This will harmonize the Spleen and Stomach.

4 Put one drop of the oil blend on each of your thumbs or index fingers and then place the oil on both the Stomach 36 points (**ST 36**). Gently massage nine small circles over each of these points. This will strengthen and harmonize the Earth element.

5 Put one drop of the oil blend on each of your thumbs or index fingers and then place the oil on both the Liver 3 points (**LV 3**)—these are Earth points on a Wood meridian. Gently massage 9 to 18 small circles over each of these points. This will calm the mind and harmonize the Liver and Spleen.

6 Lie down on your back. Place a warm moist compress on your **solar plexus**, making sure it covers the lower ribcage. Cover the compress with a dry towel and leave it in place until the compress cools.

7 Stand up and use the palm inhalation technique to inhale one drop of the oil blend.

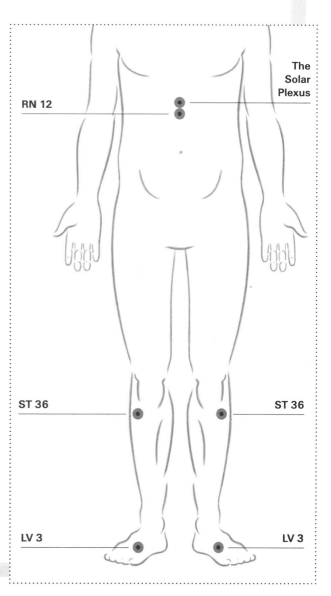

A BLEND FOR SPLEEN QI AND KIDNEY YANG DEFICIENCIES

This simple treatment can be used to stimulate and regulate digestion and warm the center.

You will need

5-ml blending bottle

Jojoba oil

2 drops ginger oil (warms the center and tonifies the Spleen and Kidney Qi)

1 drop lemongrass oil (warms the center and raises Yang)

1 drop rosemary oil (strengthens the Spleen Qi and raises Yang)

Warm moist compress (see page 52)

Towel

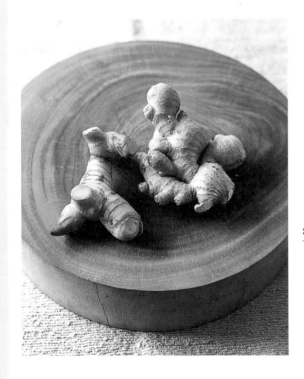

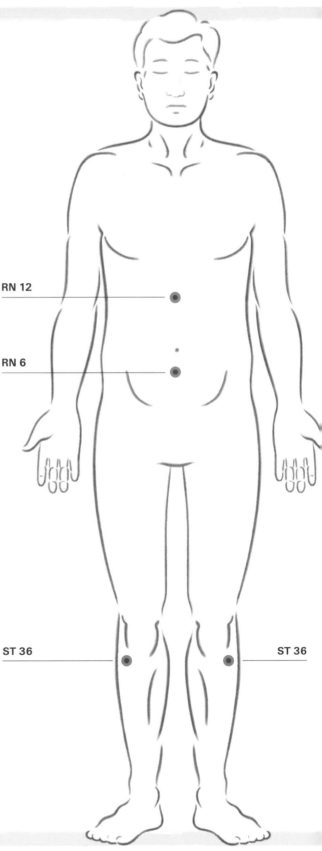

RN 12

RN 6

ST 36

ST 36

1 Fill the bottle with 1 teaspoon (5 ml) jojoba oil, then add the ginger, lemongrass, and rosemary oils and shake for a few moments.

2 Use the palm inhalation technique (see page 49) to inhale one drop of the oil blend.

3 Put one drop of the oil blend on your thumb or index finger and then place the oil on the Ren 6 point (**RN 6**). As you inhale slowly and deeply, gently but firmly press into the Ren 6 point. Hold your breath for a couple of seconds, and then exhale and release the point. Repeat nine times. This will tonify the Qi.

4 Put one drop of the oil blend on your thumb or index finger and then place the oil on the Ren 12 point (**RN 12**). Gently massage 9 to 27 small circles over the point, adding more jojoba oil if necessary. This will regulate the digestion and harmonize the Spleen.

5 Put one drop of the oil blend on each of your thumbs or index fingers and then place the oil on both the Stomach 36 points (**ST 36**). Gently massage 9 to 27 small circles over each of these points.

6 Put one drop of the oil blend on each of your thumbs or index fingers and then place the oil on the Kidney 3 point (**KD 3**) on both your legs. Gently massage nine small circles over each of these points, then massage up the Kidney meridian to the Kidney 10 point (**KD 10**) three to nine times.

7 Lie down on your back and take a few deep breaths. Place a warm moist compress on your abdomen, cover it with a dry towel, and leave it in place until the compress cools.

8 Stand up and use the palm inhalation technique to inhale one drop of the oil blend.

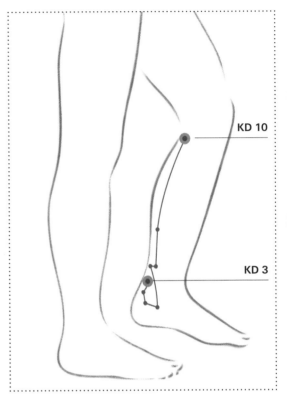

KD 10

KD 3

KEY
—•— Kidney meridian

A BLEND FOR WARMING THE CENTER

This treatment will stimulate digestion after heavy meals. It may also ease constipation.

You will need

5-ml blending bottle

Jojoba oil

3 drops sweet fennel oil (warms the center, strengthens the Kidneys, and stimulates digestion)

1 drop lemongrass oil (revives the Spleen and stimulates digestion)

1 drop ginger oil (warms the center and strengthens the Spleen and Kidneys)

Warm moist compress (see page 52)

Towel

1 Fill the bottle with 1 teaspoon (5 ml) jojoba oil, then add the sweet fennel, lemongrass, and ginger oils and shake for a few moments.
2 Put ten drops (0.5 ml) of the oil blend in the palms of your hand and then gently massage 9 to 27 clockwise circles over your abdomen from left to right.
3 Lie down on your back. Place a warm moist compress on your abdomen, cover it with a dry towel, and leave it in place until the compress cools.

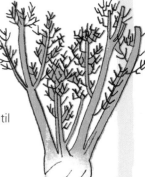

A BLEND FOR CONSTIPATION DUE TO FOOD STAGNATION

You will need

5-ml blending bottle

Jojoba oil

2 drops ginger oil (warms the center and promotes digestion)

2 drops peppermint oil (promotes the movement of Qi)

1 drop lemongrass oil (promotes the movement of Qi)

1 drop rosemary oil (strengthens and moves the Spleen Qi)

Warm moist compress (see page 52)

Towel

1 Fill the bottle with 1 teaspoon (5 ml) jojoba oil, then add the ginger, peppermint, lemongrass, and rosemary oils and shake for a few moments to combine.
2 Use the palm inhalation technique (see page 49) to inhale one drop of the oil blend.
3 Put five drops of the oil blend in the palms of your hand and then gently massage 9 to 27 circles over your abdomen, adding a little extra jojoba oil if needed.
4 Lie down on your back and take a few deep breaths. Place a warm moist compress on your lower abdomen, cover it with a dry towel, and leave it in place until the compress cools.

A BLEND TO BOOST CONFIDENCE

This treatment will strengthen Yang Qi and relieve sluggishness when digestion is not optimal. It will also help you to feel uplifted, determined, and emotionally strong.

You will need

5-ml blending bottle

Jojoba oil

2 drops sweet fennel oil (strengthens the Kidneys and stimulates Yang Qi)

1 drop basil linalool oil (warms and activates Yang Qi)

1 drop rosemary oil (warms and raises Yang Qi)

1 Fill the bottle with 1 teaspoon (5 ml) jojoba oil, then add the sweet fennel, basil, and rosemary oils and shake for a few moments.

2 Use the palm inhalation technique (see page 49) to inhale one drop of the oil blend.

3 Put one drop of the oil blend on your thumb or index finger and then place the oil on the Du 20 point (**DU 20**). Gently massage three to nine small circles over the point. This will raise Yang Qi.

4 Put one drop of the oil blend on your thumb or index finger and then place the oil on the Du 4 point (**DU 4**)—this is also known as the Ming Men point. Gently massage three to nine small circles over the point. This will strengthen both Yang Qi and the general constitution.

5 Put one drop of the oil blend on your thumb or index finger and then place the oil on the Urinary Bladder 23 point (**UB 23**). Gently massage three to nine small circles over the point. This will tonify the Kidney Qi.

6 Put one drop of the oil blend on your thumb or index finger and then place the oil on the Kidney 3 point (**KD 3**). Gently massage three to nine small circles over the point. This will tonify the Kidney Qi.

7 Use the palm inhalation technique to inhale one drop of the oil blend.

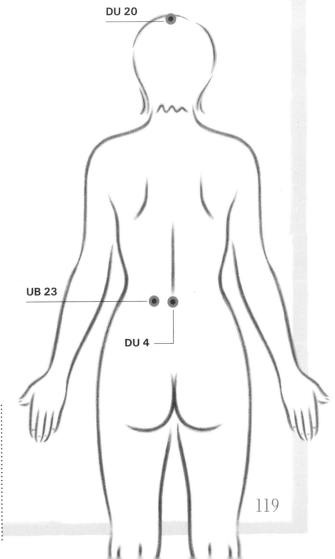

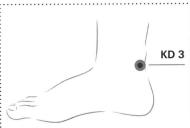

119

A BLEND FOR AROMATIC AWAKENING

This blend can be used to alleviate digestive heaviness (particularly after a very large meal) and cloudy thinking.

You will need

5-ml blending bottle

Jojoba oil

2 drops cardamom oil

2 drops peppermint oil

1 Fill the bottle with 1 teaspoon (5 ml) jojoba oil, then add the cardamom and peppermint oils and shake for a few moments.
2 Use the palm inhalation technique (see page 49) to inhale one drop of the oil blend.
3 Put one drop of the oil blend on each of your index fingers and then gently press them into the Large Intestine 20 points (**LI 20**) on either side of your face. Gently massage 9 to 27 small circles over the points.

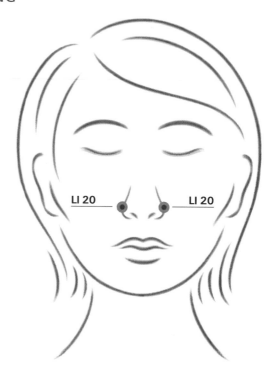

LI 20 — LI 20

....

A BLEND FOR DIGESTIVE TROUBLE DUE TO GENERAL NERVOUSNESS

This treatment is especially effective after a heavy meal.

You will need

5-ml blending bottle

Jojoba oil

2 drops neroli oil

2 drops blood orange oil

1 Fill the bottle with 1 teaspoon (5 ml) jojoba oil, then add the neroli and blood orange oils and shake for a few moments.
2 Use the palm inhalation technique (see page 49) to inhale one drop of the oil blend. Repeat three times—inhaling and exhaling nine times in total.

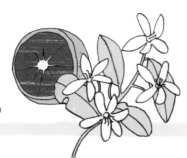

A BLEND TO BALANCE EARTH AND FIRE

This treatment can be used to nourish the spirit, relieve anxiety, and improve focus.
It may also be beneficial if you have loose stools.

You will need

5-ml blending bottle

Jojoba oil

2 drops patchouli oil (calms the mind and Heart)

1 drop neroli oil (nourishes the Blood and strengthens the Spleen)

1 drop blood orange oil (calms the Heart and supports the patchouli and neroli oils)

1 Fill the bottle with 1 teaspoon (5 ml) jojoba oil, then add the patchouli, neroli, and blood orange oils and shake for a few moments.
2 Put one drop of the oil blend on your thumb or index finger and then place the oil on the Ren 17 point (**RN 17**). Gently massage 9 to 27 small circles over the point. This will calm the Heart and influence Qi.
3 Put one drop of the oil blend on the Pericardium 6 point (**PC 6**). Using your thumb or index finger, gently massage 9 to 27 small circles over the point, then massage all the way down the Pericardium meridian to the end of the middle finger. This will calm the Shen and benefit digestion.
4 Put one drop of the oil blend on your thumb or index finger and then place the oil on the Ren 12 point (**RN 12**). Using the palm of your hand, gently massage 18 circles over the point. This will harmonize the Earth element.
5 Put one drop of the oil blend on your thumb or index finger and then place it on the Stomach 36 point (**ST 36**). Gently massage 9 to 27 small circles over the point. This will harmonize the Earth element and strengthen the Stomach and Spleen.
6 Put one drop of the oil blend on your thumb or index finger and then place it on the Spleen 3

point (**SP 3**). Gently massage the oil over the point in a circular motion. This will harmonize the Earth element and strengthens the Stomach and Spleen.

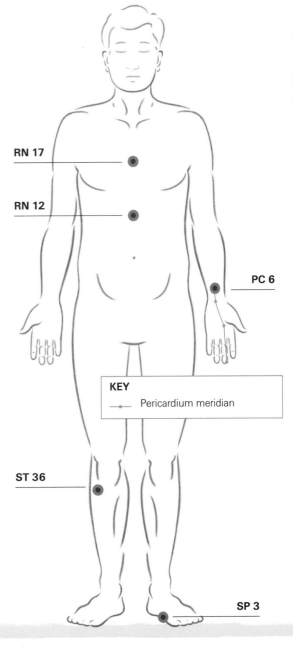

RN 17

RN 12

PC 6

KEY

Pericardium meridian

ST 36

SP 3

A TUMMY RUB TO STIMULATE SLUGGISH DIGESTION

This treatment is especially effective after a heavy meal.

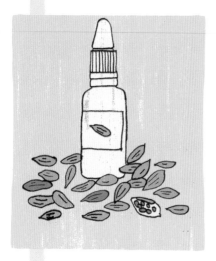

You will need

5-ml blending bottle

Jojoba oil

3 drops cardamom oil

2 drops lemon oil

Warm moist compress (see page 52)

Towel

1 Fill the bottle with 1 teaspoon (5 ml) jojoba oil, then add the cardamom and lemon oils and shake for a few moments.
2 Put ten drops (0.5 ml) of the oil blend in the palms of your hand and then gently massage 9 to 27 clockwise circles over your abdomen.
3 Lie down on your back. Place a warm moist compress on your abdomen, cover it with a dry towel, and leave it in place until the compress cools. You can repeat this step up to three times, if liked.

A MORNING PEP BLEND

This treatment aromatically opens the orifices and invigorates the senses. It is intended for those who feel sluggish and tired during the morning. It is also good for people who need a little inspiration, and it is ideal to use after overeating.

You will need

1 drop lemongrass oil

1 drop peppermint oil

1 drop Eucalyptus radiata *oil*

Cotton ball

1 Put the lemongrass, peppermint, and eucalyptus oils on a cotton ball.
2 Hold the cotton ball 3 to 4 inches (7 to 10 cm) below your nose, then gently wave the cotton ball under your nose, taking slow deep breaths.

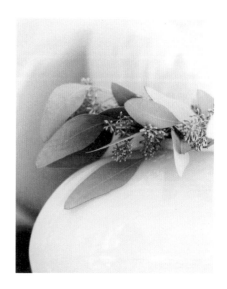

Essential Oils for Muscular Pain

Essential oils can be very beneficial to the muscular system.
This chapter will teach you about the essential oils and massage
techniques you can use to alleviate muscular pain.

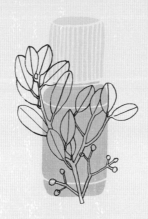

Reasons for Muscular Pain

In Chinese medicine, pain is most often associated with Qi stagnation—there is pain when there is no movement of Qi. For that reason, many of the oils that we are going to use to treat muscular pain have the ability to move Qi. Knowing which meridian or set of meridians are associated with an oil (see individual entries in Chapter 3) will help you understand where on the body that oil will move Qi.

In addition to Qi stagnation, muscular pain can also be caused by a Qi deficiency. This is a common reason for lower back pain, and it is often attributed to a Kidney Qi deficiency.

UPPER BACK PAIN

Anatomically, the layers of muscle in the upper back mostly originate at the base of the skull and then connect to the shoulder blades. For this reason, the neck and shoulders can be looked at as an enclosed system where pain in one area influences the other equally. Trauma to the tissues, stagnation in the local meridians, emotional suppression, and weakness of the body's root reserves can all create upper back pain. Pain in the upper back region, including the neck, can have a strong emotional connection.

Almost every meridian passes through this area of the body, however three of the meridians strongly influence the movement and actions of the shoulders and neck—they are the Gall Bladder, Small Intestine, and Urinary Bladder meridians.

The Gall Bladder system has a relationship with the Liver. The Liver controls the smooth flow of Qi to all areas of the body, and this dynamic process also affects the expression of emotions. In its partnership with the Liver system, the Gall Bladder controls our actions

Pain in the neck, upper shoulders, and upper back is usually interlinked.

based on our emotional and intellectual assessment. People who suffer from low energy or stagnant Gall Bladder systems can have trouble making decisions, or they can come to a decision internally but be reluctant to act.

The Gall Bladder meridian covers the sides of the entire body from the feet to the temples. Injury or stagnation in the Gall Bladder meridian can create pain or stiffness in the articulation of the shoulder joints or in the turning of the head. Those suffering from issues in this meridian may also experience headaches in the area of the temples.

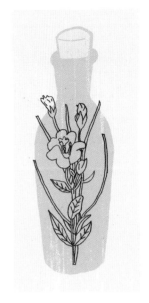

Palmarosa

The Small Intestine system pairs with the Heart. Besides controlling the flow of Blood and the vessels of the body (much as the anatomical heart), the Heart system stores the Shen (see page 27). In Chinese medicine, the Heart system is referred to as the Emperor, and—just like royalty—the Heart has influence over all the other organ systems. If one system is weak or stagnant it will affect the performance of the Heart, and thus it is afforded protection. The Small Intestine system siphons off the Heat that accumulates as a result of stressors to the Heart, and it eliminates this through urination.

The Small Intestine meridian covers the back of the arms, shoulder blades, and sides of the neck, and it ends in front of the ears. The Heart channel originates in the armpits and travels down the insides of the arms. A major influencing acupuncture point for the Heart is located on the upper back between the shoulder blades. For this reason, issues with the Small Intestine-Heart system can manifest as pain or immobility in the neck, shoulders, or elbows. This type of pattern can also occur with insomnia and/or urinary issues.

The Urinary Bladder meridian is considered one of the most superficial channels in the meridian system. Exposure to external forces such as inclement weather and extreme temperatures can easily influence this meridian. The upper part of the back and neck along the Urinary Bladder meridian are the most common areas where illness will first develop. If you've ever suffered a common cold that began with aching pain and stiffness along the back of the neck and the base of the skull, you've likely experienced the situation of a pathogen affecting the Urinary Bladder meridian.

Common oils that are beneficial for the upper back and neck pain are palmarosa, *Eucalyptus radiata*, *Eucalyptus globulus*, basil, rosemary, tea tree, ravensara, and sweet marjoram.

MIDDLE BACK PAIN

Pain and tension in the middle of the back is often associated with a tug-of-war between the Liver and Spleen. A deficiency of the Spleen-Stomach can create a weak spot where the energies of the Liver become hyperactive. This imbalance between the two systems has a strong effect on emotional expression, leading to irritability, reactivity, and angry outbursts.

Another important connection in this area of the body is the exchange between the Lungs and the Liver. The Lungs are the pacemakers for many areas of the body. Our pattern of inhalation and exhalation moves the diaphragm to massage the Liver, which in turn massages the Intestines. In a healthy individual, this process engenders emotional calm and supports digestion and motility of the gut to remove waste. In a situation of stress or imbalance, respiration may be incomplete or too shallow to engage in this self-supporting cycle. In such a scenario, anxiety and irritability arise, the gut slows down, and the muscles of the middle back become hyper-engaged. People who experience this often describe it as a feeling of wearing a tight belt around their midsection. As this imbalance becomes advanced, the overuse of the mid-back can contribute to a weakened lower back.

The essential oils that have an effect on the middle back all have affinities to the Lungs, Liver, and Spleen. Lavender, Roman chamomile, sweet marjoram, lemongrass, rosemary, ravensara, and tea tree are common oils that are used to treat middle back pain.

Middle back pain can be caused by tension between the organs in this area.

LOWER BACK PAIN

The lower back can be seen as an area of foundation for the body. The lumbar area and the hips sustain a lot of the body's weight, and they must remain flexible but strong to keep us upright. The two main damaging influences on this area of the body are weakness of the Kidney system and stagnation in the Gall Bladder meridian.

As discussed earlier in this section (see page 124), the Gall Bladder meridian passes along the sides of the entire body. This includes connecting internally to and facilitating articulation of the joints of the ankles, knees, hips, and shoulders. The Gall Bladder meridian has a strong connection to the ease of movement in the hip joint and the muscles surrounding that area. Stagnation or deficiency along the meridian in this area can manifest as stiffness or pain of the hip joint.

The Kidney system houses the body's energy reserves (see page 25) and influences bone health. For these reasons, issues of the spine, especially in the lumbar area, can be connected to the Kidney system. Weakness of the lower back and knees can often be a reflection of a deficiency of the Kidney system. The Kidneys also support healthy sexual function and reproduction. Issues with fertility, libido, and sexual performance can all be the result of a weakened Kidney system, especially when occurring along with pain, weakness, or immobility of the lower back.

The essential oils that have an effect on the lower back all have an affinity to the Kidneys. Most of these oils are warming—tea tree being the most notable exception to this rule. Essential oils that are beneficial for the lower back include ginger, Scots pine, lemongrass, vetiver, and sweet marjoram.

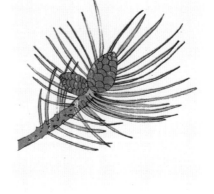

Scots pine

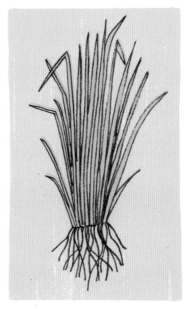

Vetiver

BI SYNDROME

Bi syndrome is the name for a pattern of blockage that can occur anywhere in the body. Stuffed sinuses are referred to as a Nasal Bi, and coronary heart disease might be classified as a Chest Bi in most instances. However, Bi syndrome is most common in the joints. As the meridian system covers the entire body, the multifaceted articulations of the joints become a vulnerable area prone to stagnation, and thus pain and disease.

Bi syndrome affecting the joints has several classifications based on its characteristic presentation. These classifications help us to choose the most appropriate course of treatment. However, it is important to note that almost every Bi pattern is multisided. It is almost unheard of to find a presentation that is only one classification, rather most have combinations of multiple types with one or two main characteristics. For this reason, many of the essential oils that are going to benefit one category's symptoms will also aid in another.

Types of Bi Pattern

Wind Bi

Wind (see page 37) is identified by its traveling nature. In this presentation, pain moves from one side of the joint to the other, jumps the sides of the body, and to other joints. This type of Bi is often accompanied by numbness or itching.

Damp Bi

Damp (see page 37) is known for its strongly stagnant nature. Dampness stays fixed in its location, never traveling. This type of Bi can be accompanied by a sensation of heaviness or pressure.

Cold Bi

Cold (see page 37) is contracting and stagnating in nature, and it gives rise to pain. This type of pain is characterized by being worse in cold weather and soothed with a heat pad or warm bath. Cold Bi is also associated with stiffness that is worse at rest and loosens up with mild activity.

Hot Bi

The type of Bi is accompanied by sharp pains, redness, swelling, and a sensation of heat in the affected joint. Hot Bi is an uncomfortable condition that can be soothed by the application of cold.

Base Oils for Muscle and Joint Pain

We need to use base oils to dilute essential oils before we apply them to the skin (see page 51). Some base oils can benefit certain conditions. For example, arnica and sesame oils are good for muscular and joint pain.

ARNICA

Arnica *(Arnica montana)* is known for its unique anti-inflammatory, soothing, and healing properties. It is often used for traumatic injuries to the muscles, joints, and ligaments, and it can also be used to relax muscles after workouts, and to reduce bruising.

Arnica is grown in the mountainous regions of Europe and Siberia. It has been an important medicinal plant in these regions since the fifteenth century, and it is still popular in herbal medicine today. Due to its proven efficacy, arnica is included in the herbal pharmacopoeias of several countries, including Germany, the United Kingdom, and the USA. Arnica is often used in pain-relieving creams, gels, ointments, and oils.

Arnica oil should be used as 10 to 20 percent of an oil blend.

SESAME OIL

Sesame oil is an edible vegetable oil derived from sesame seeds. It is a very popular cooking oil in southern India, and it is often used as a flavor enhancer in Chinese, Japanese, Middle Eastern, Korean, and Southeast Asian cuisine.

Sesame oil is easily absorbed into the skin, and it has analgesic properties.

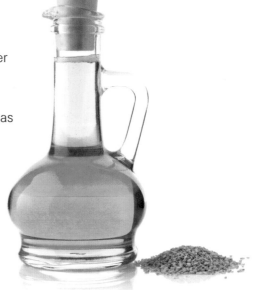

Sesame oil

Blends to Ease Muscular Aches and Pains

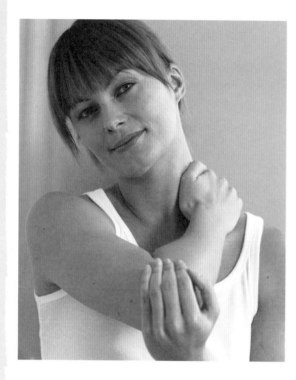

A BLEND TO RELEASE UPPER NECK AND TRAPEZIUS PAIN

You will need

60 drops (3 ml) arnica oil

9 drops sweet marjoram oil

6 drops lavender oil

5 drops peppermint oil

½ fl oz (15-ml) blending bottle

Jojoba oil

*2 warm moist compresses (see page 52)—
the first compress is optional (see step 2)*

Towel

1 Put the arnica, sweet marjoram, lavender, and peppermint oils in the bottle, then top it off with jojoba oil and shake for a few moments.

2 (This step is optional, but may prove beneficial.) Apply a warm moist compress to the painful area of your neck, cover it with a dry towel, and hold it in place until the compress cools.

3 Put 10 to 20 drops of the oil blend in the palms of your hand and then massage the tender areas of your neck for 3 to 8 minutes.

4 Apply a warm moist compress to the painful area of your neck, cover it with a dry towel, and hold it in place until the compress cools.

USING LEMONGRASS TO RELIEVE HIP PAIN AND SCIATICA RELIEF

Blend 1

You will need

15 drops (0.75 ml) jojoba or arnica oil

3 drops lemongrass oil

1. Put the jojoba or arnica oil in the palms of your hand and then add the lemongrass oil. Massage the oil over your lower back and hip in a downward fashion.

Blend 2

You will need

10-ml blending bottle

Jojoba oil

12 drops lemongrass oil

1. Fill the bottle with 2 teaspoons (10 ml) jojoba oil, then add the lemongrass oil and shake for a few moments.
2. Put two to three drops of the oil blend on your thumb or index finger and then place the oil on the Gall Bladder 34 point (**GB 34**). Firmly massage nine small circles over the point.
3. Put two to three drops of the oil blend on your thumb or index finger and then place the oil on the Gall Bladder 41 point (**GB 41**). Gently massage nine small circles over the point.
4. Put two to three drops of the oil blend on your thumb or index finger and then place the oil on the Liver 3 point (**LV 3**). Gently massage nine small circles over the point.
5. Put two to three drops of the oil blend on your thumb or index finger and then place the oil on the Urinary Bladder 18 point (**UB 18**). Gently massage nine small circles over the point.

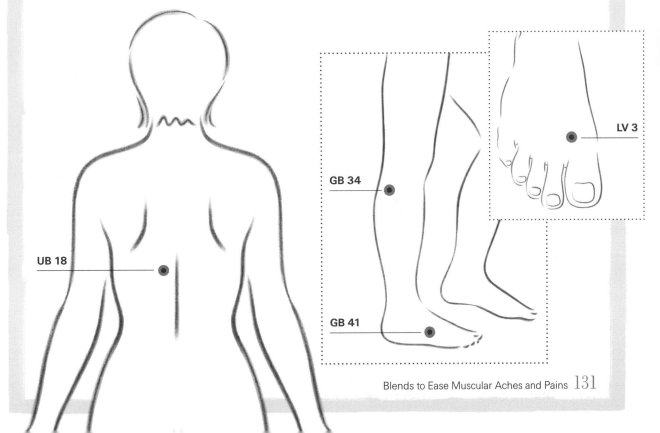

GB 34

LV 3

UB 18

GB 41

A BLEND TO PROMOTE THE MOVEMENT OF LIVER QI

This blend is beneficial for pain along the sides of the ribs, hips, and the outside of the legs. It also relieves a sense of being stuck.

You will need

5-ml blending bottle

Jojoba oil

2 drops lemongrass oil (promotes the movement of Liver Qi and relaxes the muscles)

2 drops lavender oil (promotes the movement of Liver Qi and calms the Shen)

1 drop peppermint oil (spreads Liver Qi)

Warm moist compress (see page 52)

Towel

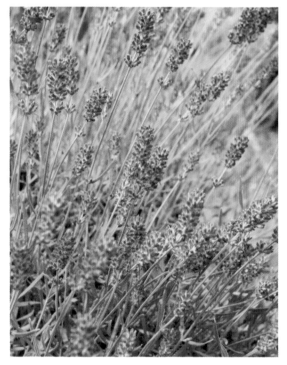

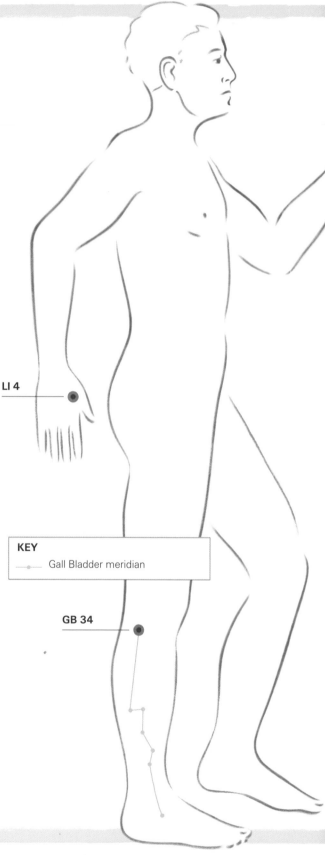

LI 4

KEY

Gall Bladder meridian

GB 34

1. Fill the bottle with 1 teaspoon (5 ml) jojoba oil, then add the lemongrass, lavender, and peppermint oils and shake for a few moments.
2. Put one drop of the oil blend on the Large Intestine 4 point (**LI 4**). Using your thumb or index finger, gently massage 9 to 27 small circles over the point.
3. Put one drop of the oil blend on your thumb or index finger and then place the oil on the Liver 3 point (**LV 3**). Gently massage 9 to 27 small circles over the point.
4. Put one drop of the oil blend on your thumb or index finger and then place the oil on the Gall Bladder 34 point (**GB 34**). Gently massage 9 to 27 small circles over the point, then massage down the Gall Bladder meridian to the ankle three to nine times.
5. Put one drop of the oil blend on your thumb or index finger and then place the oil on your **solar plexus**.
6. Put 15 drops (0.75 ml) jojoba oil in the palm of your hand and then gently massage the oil into your solar plexus in large circular motions.
7. Lie down on your back. Place a warm moist compress on your solar plexus, cover it with a dry towel, and leave it in place until the compress cools. You can repeat this step up to three times, if liked.

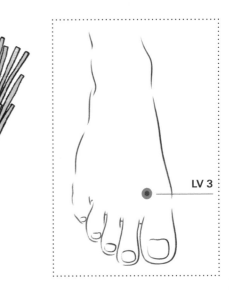

LV 3

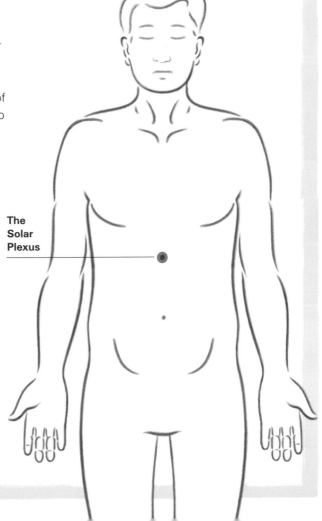

The Solar Plexus

A BLEND TO HARMONIZE THE LIVER AND SPLEEN

This treatment promotes calmness and relaxation. It is beneficial for irritability, frustration, pain along the side of the ribs, abdominal bloating, indigestion, muscle pain, alternating loose stools and constipation, and difficulty making decisions.

You will need

5-ml blending bottle

Jojoba oil

1 drop lavender oil (calms the Shen)

1 drop Roman chamomile oil (soothes the Liver, calms the Shen, and harmonizes the Liver and Spleen)

1 drop peppermint oil (spreads Liver Qi)

1 drop bergamot oil (calms the Shen)

1 drop lemongrass oil (moves Liver Qi and harmonizes the Liver and Spleen)

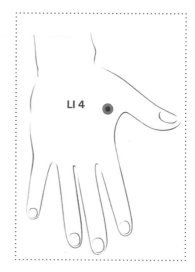

1 Fill the bottle with 1 teaspoon (5 ml) jojoba oil, then add the lavender, Roman chamomile, peppermint, bergamot, and lemongrass oils and shake for a few moments.

2 Use the palm inhalation technique (see page 49) to inhale one drop of the oil blend.

3 Put one drop of the oil blend on the Large Intestine 4 point (**LI 4**) on one of your hands. Using your thumb or index finger, gently massage the oil over the point in a circular motion for a few seconds. Repeat on the Large Intestine 4 point on the other hand. This promotes the movement of Qi.

4 Put one drop of the oil blend on each of your thumbs or index fingers and then place the oil on the Liver 3 point (**LV 3**) on both your feet. Gently massage the oil over the points in a circular motion for a few seconds. This promotes the movement of Qi.

5 Put one drop of the oil blend on your thumb or index finger and then place the oil on the Spleen 3 point (**SP 3**). Gently massage the oil over the point in a circular motion for a few seconds.

6 Put one drop of the oil blend on your thumb or index finger and then place the oil on the Stomach 36 point (**ST 36**). Gently massage the oil over the point in a circular motion for a few seconds.

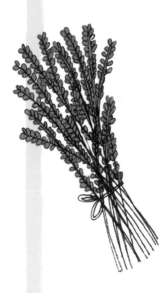

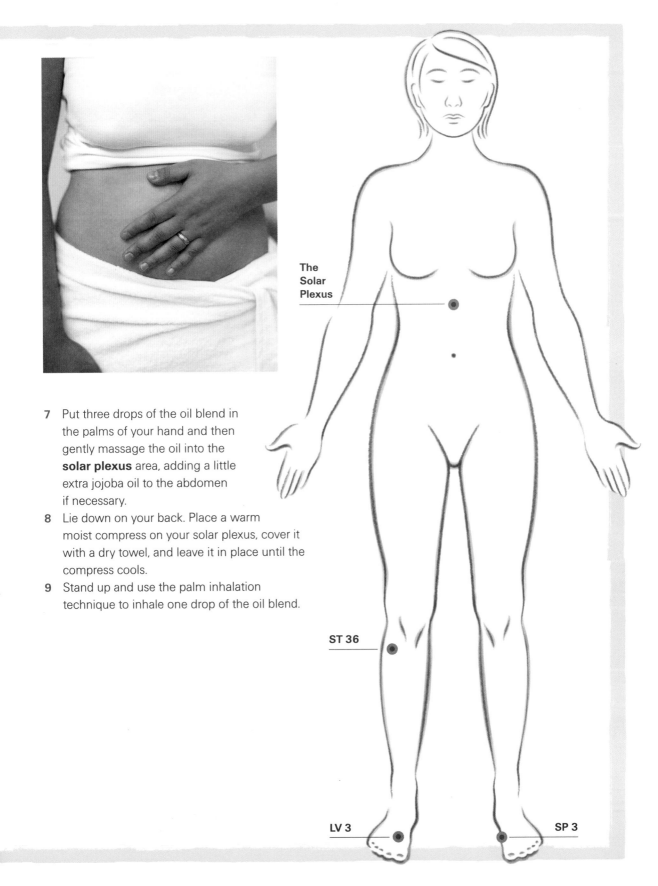

The
Solar
Plexus

7   Put three drops of the oil blend in
    the palms of your hand and then
    gently massage the oil into the
    solar plexus area, adding a little
    extra jojoba oil to the abdomen
    if necessary.

8   Lie down on your back. Place a warm
    moist compress on your solar plexus, cover it
    with a dry towel, and leave it in place until the
    compress cools.

9   Stand up and use the palm inhalation
    technique to inhale one drop of the oil blend.

ST 36

LV 3

SP 3

A BATH TO HELP YOU BE HERE NOW

These two scented baths will help to strengthen the Lungs and relax the muscles.

You will need

Small bowl

2 to 3 tablespoons (30 to 45 ml) liquid Castile soap (or you can use vegetable or jojoba oil)

Blend 1

2 drops Scots pine oil

2 drops lavender oil

2 drops tea tree oil

Blend 2

2 drops Scots pine oil

2 drops Eucalyptus radiata oil

2 drops ravensara oil

1 Mix together the soap and your chosen blend of essential oils in a small bowl.
2 Fill a bathtub with hot water, then add the soap mixture and swirl to mix well.
3 Get into the bath and soak in the water for about 20 minutes.

A BLEND TO RELIEVE A BACK WITH A DULL ACHE

This treatment will strengthen the Kidneys and willpower.

You will need

½ fl oz (15-ml) blending bottle

Jojoba oil

8 drops Scots pine oil (tonifies the Kidney Qi)

6 drops tea tree oil (tonifies the Kidney Qi)

2 drops ginger oil (strengthens the Kidneys and warms the lower back)

2 drops sweet marjoram oil (relaxes the muscles)

Warm moist compress (see page 52)

Large plastic bag (it needs to be large enough to hold the compress)

1 Fill the bottle with 3 teaspoons (15 ml) jojoba oil, then add the Scots pine, tea tree, ginger, and sweet marjoram oils and shake for a few moments.
2 Put 10 drops (0.5 ml) of the oil blend in the palms of your hand and then gently massage your lower back in a circular motion for three to five minutes.
3 Place a warm moist compress in a plastic bag. Lie down on your back with the bag-wrapped compress positioned under your lower back. Remain in this position until the compress cools.

A BLEND TO RELIEVE JOINT PAIN DUE TO COLD

This treatment uses warmth and movement to alleviate pain. It is particularly beneficial for Wind-Damp-Cold Bi and Cold-Damp Bi. The massage can be done twice per day. The regimen should be performed six days in a row, followed by one day off. Alternatively, it can be done three days on, one day off, and then three days on again. If this massage is being used to relieve pain in the ankles, add four drops of vetiver or myrrh oil to the blend.

You will need

60 drops (3 ml) sesame oil

60 drops (3 ml) arnica oil

4 drops lavender oil (balances out the warming oils in the blend and circulates Qi)

3 drops Eucalyptus globulus oil (warms the meridians and alleviates muscular aches and joint pains, especially those in the upper body)

3 drops ginger oil (warms and opens the meridians, invigorates the Blood, and stops pain, especially pain in the hips and lower body)

3 drops lemongrass oil (promotes the movement of Qi and relaxes sinews and ligaments)

3 drops frankincense oil (invigorates the Blood, reduces inflammation, and alleviates pain)

3 drops Scots pine oil (strengthens the Kidneys, increases circulation, and alleviates pain)

3 drops ravensara oil (alleviates pain)

½ fl oz (15-ml) blending bottle

Jojoba oil

Warm moist compress (see page 52)

Towel

1. Put the sesame, arnica, lavender, eucalyptus, ginger, lemongrass, frankincense, Scots pine, and ravensara oils in the bottle, then top it off with jojoba oil (about 1½ teaspoons/8 ml) and shake for a few moments.
2. Apply a warm moist compress to the painful area, cover it with a dry towel, and hold it in place for a few minutes.
3. Put 20 drops (1 ml) of the oil blend in the palms of your hand and then gently massage the painful area for one to three minutes.
4. Apply a warm moist compress to the painful area and cover it with a dry towel. After about 15 seconds, begin to very gently flex, extend, and rotate the joint until the compress cools. Repeat up to three times.

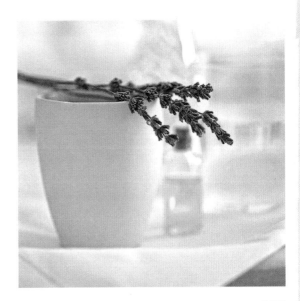

A BLEND TO RELIEVE JOINT PAIN DUE TO HEAT

This blend will alleviate pain and reduce inflammation. It is particularly beneficial for Hot-Damp Bi. The massage can be done twice per day. The regimen should be performed six days in a row, followed by one day off. Alternatively, it can be done three days on, one day off, and then three days on again.

You will need

60 drops (3 ml) sesame oil

60 drops (3 ml) arnica oil

6 drops palmarosa oil (cools, clears Heat, and reduces inflammation)

4 drops frankincense oil (cools, invigorates the Blood, reduces inflammation, and alleviates pain)

3 drops lavender oil (cools, clears Heat, and reduces inflammation)

3 drops Roman chamomile oil (clears heat, reduces inflammation, and alleviates pain)

3 drops peppermint oil (cools and alleviates pain)

3 drops vetiver oil (stimulates the circulation, reduces inflammation, and alleviates pain)

½ fl oz (15-ml) blending bottle

Jojoba oil

Warm moist compress (see page 52)

Towel

1 Put the sesame, arnica, palmarosa, frankincense, lavender, Roman chamomile, peppermint, and vetiver oils in the bottle, then top it off with jojoba oil (about 1½ teaspoons/ 8 ml) and shake for a few moments.
2 Apply a warm moist compress to the painful area, cover it with a dry towel, and hold it in place for a few minutes.
3 Put 20 drops (1 ml) of the oil blend in the palms of your hand and then gently massage the painful area for one to three minutes.
4 Apply a warm moist compress to the painful area and cover it with a dry towel. After about 15 seconds, begin to very gently flex, extend, and rotate the joint until the compress cools. Repeat up to three times.

- -

USING PEPPERMINT FOR A TEMPORAL HEADACHE

You will need

5-ml blending bottle

Jojoba oil

8 to 10 drops peppermint oil

1 Fill the bottle with 1 teaspoon (5 ml) jojoba oil, then add the peppermint oil and shake for a few moments.
2 Use the palm inhalation technique (see page 49) to inhale one drop of the oil blend.
3 Put two drops of the oil blend on each of your index fingers and then place the oil on your temples. Using the first three fingers on each hand, gently massage the oil into your temples in a circular motion, being careful not to let the oil touch your eyes.

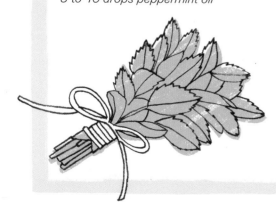

Chapter

7

Essential Oils for General Relaxation

In this chapter, we are going to focus on calming and relaxing the mind. Or in other words, calming the Shen (see page 27). A lot of the blends we will use include middle or base note oils that work well for symptoms of anxiety, restlessness, and insomnia.

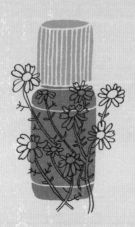

Causes of Stress

In modern life we are well acquainted with shouldering a daily dose of stress. Often we think that we need more energy and more willpower in order to be successful, but this common view that the path to the top is only through hard work ignores our body's (and our mind's) need for rest in order to perform optimally.

Many of us don't understand what our bodies need. In the face of our stressful day-to-day lives, often we turn to various coping mechanisms, instead of trying to achieve true rest. Smoking, drinking coffee and/or alcohol, sexual activity, overeating, and the intake of recreational substances are common ways that many of us use to vent stress and promote relaxation. While we don't want to do away with all the fun things in life, it is important to recognize that such coping activities impact our bodies in much the same ways as the stressors we are trying to avoid.

Many of us are stuck in a cycle of depleting our energy stores (see page 23) through overwork and stress, and then further depleting them through our recreational activities. This cycle results in lowered organ function, the imbalance of hormone secretions, and the suppression of emotions. In turn, this lowered function leads to poor waste elimination, not only in terms of urine and stools but also in the removal of metabolic wastes from the cells to make room for new nutrients.

People who need to repair their bodies through relaxation often have difficulty in identifying and/or expressing their feelings. They may feel controlled by a particular emotion or a narrative about a past injustice or trauma.

Essential oils act directly on the limbic system, the part of the brain that regulates much of our emotional landscape and our base responses to stressors such as fear. In this way, essential oils are key to working through our behavioral adaptations to stress, and moving us to a place of true rest and rehabilitation.

Blends for Relaxation

A DIFFUSION TO IMPROVE FOCUS

When we are stressed, our focus may suffer. This blend can help.

You will need

Candle, mist, or electric diffuser

2 drops peppermint oil

1 drop basil oil

1 drop rosemary cineole oil

1 Fill the diffuser with water and then add the peppermint, basil, and rosemary oils.
2 Light the candle or turn on the diffuser.

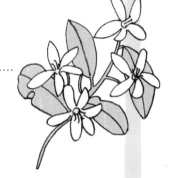

A BLEND TO CALM SPIRIT

Blood orange and neroli both aid in calming the spirit and mind, especially if there are frustrations and agitations that are keeping you from feel joy and happiness. Set your intention to feel joy.

You will need

5-ml blending bottle

Jojoba oil

2 drops blood orange oil

2 drops neroli oil

1 Fill the bottle with 1 teaspoon (5 ml) jojoba oil, then add the blood orange and neroli oils and shake for a few moments.
2 Use the palm inhalation technique (see page 49) to inhale one drop of the oil blend.

TRANQUILITY BATH

This meditative bath will help to ease nerves and calm the mind.

You will need

Small bowl

2 to 3 tablespoons (30 to 45 ml) liquid Castile soap (or you can use vegetable or jojoba oil)

2 drops geranium oil

2 drops palmarosa oil

2 drops sandalwood oil

1 Mix together the soap and essential oils in a small bowl.
2 Fill a bathtub with hot water, then add the soap mixture and swirl to mix well.
3 Get into the bath and soak in the water for about 20 minutes.

USING LAVENDER FOR STRESS RELIEF

This treatment can be used whenever you feel mildly frustrated or irritated—at home, at work, or even stuck in traffic. For a quick version of this treatment, omit step five. If you would like a more uplifting effect, you can add one drop of peppermint oil to the blend.

You will need

5-ml blending bottle

Jojoba oil

3 drops lavender oil

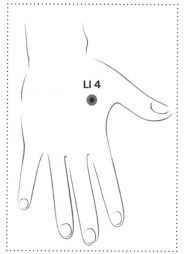

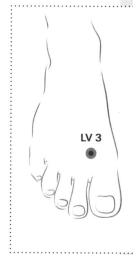

1 Fill the bottle with 1 teaspoon (5 ml) jojoba oil, then add the lavender oil and shake for a few moments.

2 Use the palm inhalation technique (see page 49) to inhale one drop of the oil blend.

3 Put one drop of the oil blend on the Large Intestine 4 point (**LI 4**) on one of your hands. Using your thumb or index finger, gently massage the oil over the point in a circular motion for a few seconds. Repeat on the Large Intestine 4 point on the other hand. This promotes the movement of Qi.

4 Put one drop of the oil blend on each of your thumbs or index fingers and then place the oil on the Liver 3 point (**LV 3**) on both your feet. Gently massage the oil over the points in a circular motion for a few seconds. This promotes the movement of Qi.

5 Put one drop of the oil blend on your thumb or index finger and then place the oil on the Du 24 point (**DU 24**), being careful not to let the oil touch your eyes or eyebrows. Gently massage the oil over the point for a few seconds.

6 Use the palm inhalation technique to inhale one drop of the oil blend.

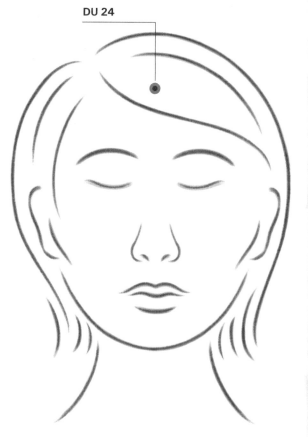

A BLEND FOR DEEP AND MEANINGFUL RELAXATION

This treatment encourages a deep sense of calm, and is especially beneficial if performed before the start of a massage.

You will need

5-ml blending bottle

Jojoba oil

3 drops vetiver oil

1 Fill the bottle with 1 teaspoons (5ml) jojoba oil, then add the vetiver oil and shake for a few moments.

2 Put one drop of the oil blend on your thumb or index finger and then place the oil on the Kidney 1 point (**KD 1**). Gently massage three to nine small circles over the point.

3 Put one drop of the oil blend on your thumb or index finger and then place the oil on the Urinary Bladder 23 point (**UB 23**). Gently massage three to nine small circles over the point.

4 Put one drop of the oil blend on your thumb or index finger and then place the oil on the Urinary Bladder 15 point (**UB 15**). Gently massage three to nine small circles over the point.

5 Put one drop of the oil blend on your thumb or index finger and then place the oil on the Du 14 point (**DU 14**). Gently massage three to nine small circles over the point.

6 Use the palm inhalation technique (see page 49) to inhale one drop of the oil blend.

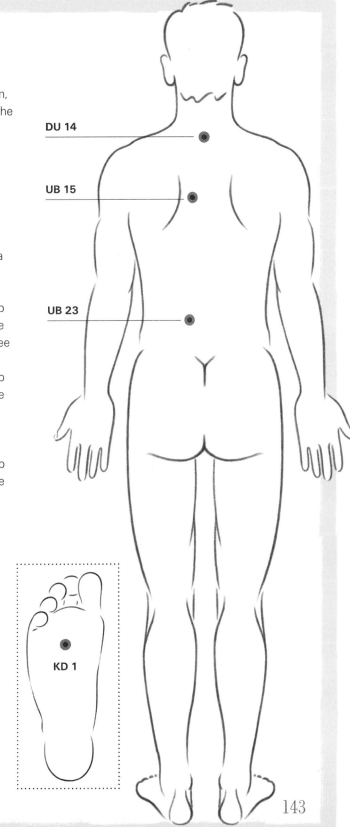

DU 14

UB 15

UB 23

KD 1

143

SIMPLE CALMING WITH GERANIUM

You will need

5-ml blending bottle

Jojoba oil

3 drops geranium oil

1 Fill the bottle with 1 teaspoon (5 ml) jojoba oil, then add the geranium oil and shake for a few moments.
2 Use the palm inhalation technique (see page 49) to inhale one drop of the oil blend.
3 Put one drop of the oil blend on your thumb or index finger and then place the oil on the Du 24 point (**DU 24**), being careful not to let the oil touch your eyes or eyebrows. Gently massage 9 to 27 small circles over the point.
4 Put one drop of the oil blend on your thumb and then place the oil on the **Yintang** point, being careful not to let the oil touch your eyes or eyebrows. Gently massage 9 to 27 small circles over the point.
5 Use the palm inhalation technique to inhale one drop of the oil blend.

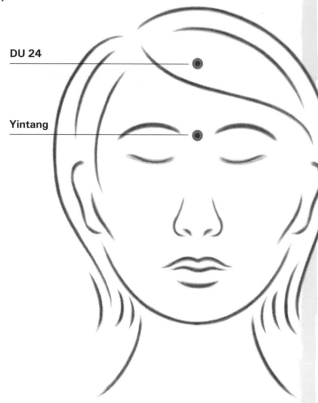

DU 24

Yintang

A BATH TO NOURISH THE HEART

This gentle and cooling bath can be used to promote relaxation and calmness.

You will need

Small bowl

2 to 3 tablespoons (30 to 45 ml) liquid Castile soap (or you can use vegetable or jojoba oil)

2 drops geranium oil (calms the mind, relaxes the Heart, and promotes rest)

1 drop lavender oil (calms the mind and Heart and promotes a sense of relaxation)

1 drop bergamot oil (uplifts and relaxes)

1 Mix together the soap and essential oils in a small bowl.
2 Fill a bathtub with hot water, then add the soap mixture and swirl to mix well.
3 Get into the bath and soak in the water for about 20 minutes.

A SOOTHING NIGHTTIME BATH

This aromatic bath is beneficial for nervousness and sleeplessness. It's ideal if you are apprehensive about a situation on the following day. This bath will open the Heart and calm the Shen.

You will need

Small bowl

2 to 3 tablespoons (30 to 45 ml) liquid Castile soap (or you can use vegetable or jojoba oil)

2 drops frankincense oil

2 drops geranium oil

2 drops sandalwood oil

2 drops lavender oil

1 Mix together the soap and essential oils in a small bowl.
2 Fill a bathtub with hot water, then add the soap mixture and swirl to mix well.
3 Get into the bath and soak in the water for about 20 minutes.

SIMPLE CALMING WITH GERMAN CHAMOMILE

You will need

5-ml blending bottle

Jojoba oil

1 drop German chamomile oil

1 Fill the bottle with 1 teaspoon (5 ml) jojoba oil, then add the German chamomile oil and shake for a few moments.
2 Put one drop of the oil blend on each of your thumbs or index fingers and then place the oil on the Kidney 1 point (**KD 1**) on both your feet. Gently massage the oil over the points for 30 seconds to 3 minutes.

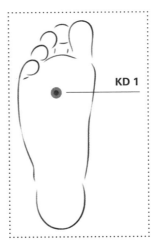

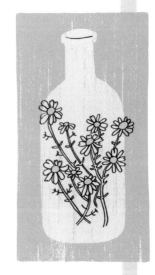

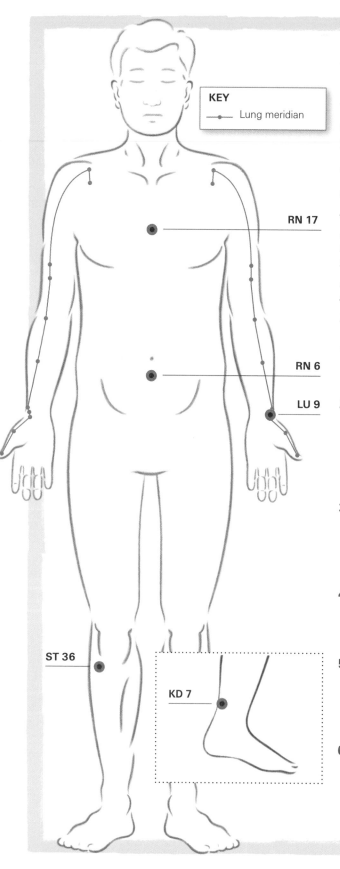

RN 17

RN 6

LU 9

ST 36

KD 7

A BLEND TO HELP YOU MOVE FORWARD

This blend helps to release longings for the past so that you are able to be in the present and move forward.

You will need

5-ml blending bottle

Jojoba oil

2 drops frankincense oil (increases depth of respiration, allows for forgiveness and taking in new life)

2 drops geranium oil (nourishes the Heart and allows for forgiveness)

2 drops rosemary oil (tonifies the Heart Qi)

1 Fill the bottle with 1 teaspoon (5 ml) jojoba oil, then add the frankincense, geranium, and rosemary oils and shake for a few moments.

2 Put one drop of the oil blend on the Lung 9 point (**LU 9**). Using your thumb or index finger, gently massage one to three small circles over the point, then massage all the way up and down the Lung meridian nine times. This will tonify the Lung Qi.

3 Put one drop of the oil blend on your thumb or index finger and then place the oil on the Ren 17 point (**RN 17**). Gently massage nine small circles over the point. This will open the chest and influence Qi.

4 Put one drop of the oil blend on your thumb or index finger and then place the oil on the Ren 6 point (**RN 6**). Gently massage nine small circles over the point. This will tonify the Qi.

5 Put one drop of the oil blend on your thumb or index finger and then place the oil on the Stomach 36 point (**ST 36**). Gently massage nine small circles over the point. This will tonify the Qi.

6 Put one drop of the oil blend on your thumb or index finger and then place the oil on the Kidney 7 point (**KD 7**). Gently massage nine small circles over the point. This will tonify the Lung and Kidney Qi.

CONTEMPLATIVE MEDITATION

You will need

5-ml blending bottle

Jojoba oil

3 drops sandalwood oil

1 Fill the bottle with 1 teaspoon (5 ml) jojoba oil, then add the sandalwood oil and shake for a few moments.

2 Sit in a comfortable position with your spine straight.

3 Use the palm inhalation technique (see page 49) to inhale one drop of the oil blend. Repeat three times—inhaling and exhaling nine times in total.

4 Put one drop of the oil blend on your thumb or index finger and then place the oil on the **Yintang** point, being careful not to let the oil touch your eyes or eyebrows. Gently massage nine small circles over the point.

5 Put one drop of the oil blend on your thumb or index finger and then place the oil on the Ren 17 point (**RN 17**). Gently massage the oil over the point with small circular motions.

6 Put one drop of the oil blend on your thumb or index finger and then place the oil on the Ren 6 point (**RN 6**). Gently massage nine small circles over the point.

7 Put one drop of the oil blend on your thumb or index finger and then place the oil on the Kidney 3 point (**KD 3**). Gently massage nine small circles over the point.

8 Use the palm inhalation technique to inhale one drop of the oil blend. Repeat three times—inhaling and exhaling nine times in total.

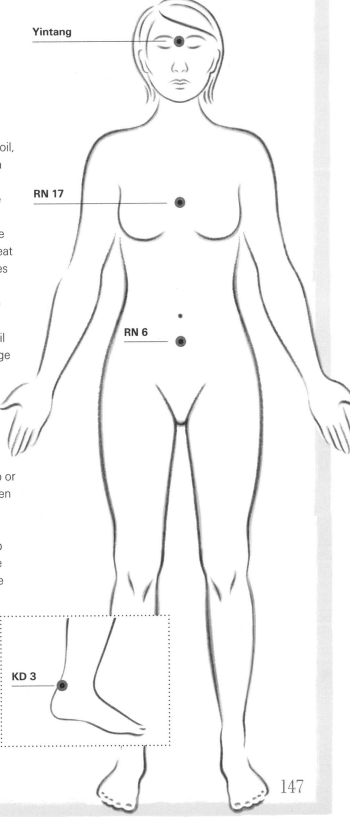

USING PALMAROSA TO INVITE CALM AND RELAXATION

Palmarosa has an affinity with the energetic points used in this massage.
If you prefer, you can substitute geranium oil for palmarosa oil.

You will need

5-ml blending bottle

Jojoba oil

3 drops palmarosa oil

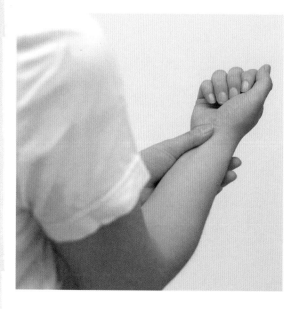

1 Fill the bottle with 1 teaspoon (5 ml) jojoba oil, then add the palmarosa oil and shake for a few moments.

2 Put one drop of the oil blend on your thumb or index finger and then place the oil on the Du 24 point (**DU 24**), being careful not to let the oil touch your eyes or eyebrows. Gently massage in small circles from the point toward the midpoint of the head three times.

3 Put one drop of the oil blend on your thumb or index finger and then place the oil on the **Yintang** point, being careful not to let the oil touch your eyes or eyebrows. Gently massage three small circles over the point.

4 Put one drop of the oil blend on your thumb or index finger and then place the oil on the Ren 17 point (**RN 17**). Gently massage three small circles over the point.

5 Put two drops of the oil blend on the Pericardium 6 point (**PC 6**). Using your thumb or index finger, gently massage the oil over the point in slow circular motions and then massage down the meridian to the Pericardium 8 point (**PC 8**) three times. Massage the Pericardium 8 point in a circular motion.

6 Put one drop of the oil blend on your thumb or index finger and then place the oil on the Liver 3 point (**LV 3**). Gently massage over the point with slow circular motions.

7 Use the palm inhalation technique (see page 49) to inhale one drop of the oil blend.

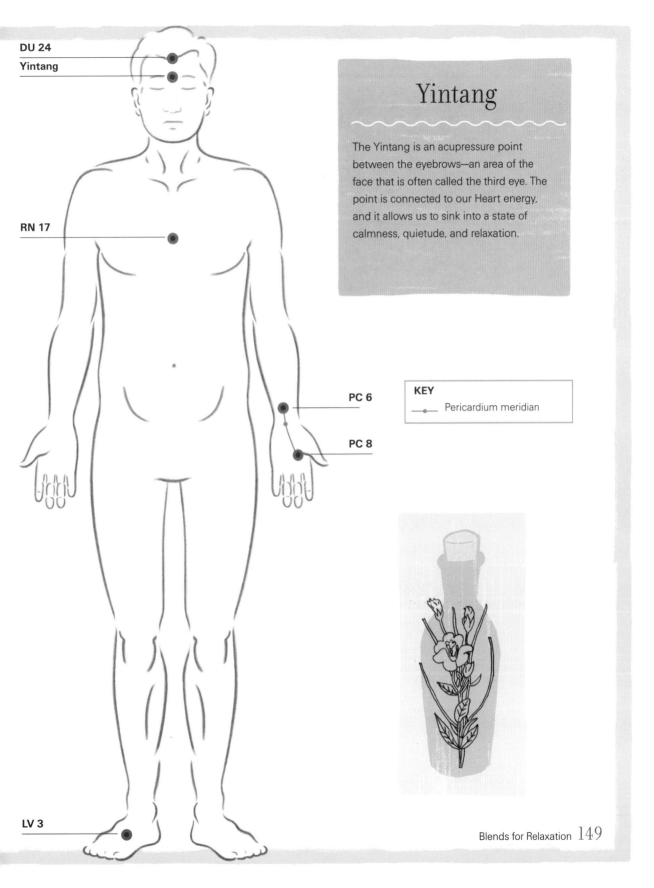

DU 24

Yintang

RN 17

Yintang

The Yintang is an acupressure point between the eyebrows—an area of the face that is often called the third eye. The point is connected to our Heart energy, and it allows us to sink into a state of calmness, quietude, and relaxation.

PC 6

PC 8

KEY
— Pericardium meridian

LV 3

OPENING HEART MEDITATION

You will need

5-ml blending bottle

Jojoba oil

3 drops sandalwood oil

1 drop geranium or palmarosa oil

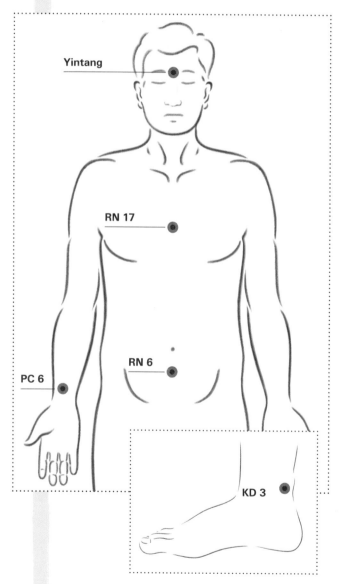

1 Fill the bottle with 1 teaspoon (5 ml) jojoba oil, then add the sandalwood and geranium or palmarosa oils and shake for a few moments.

2 Sit in a comfortable position with your spine straight.

3 Use the palm inhalation technique (see page 49) to inhale one drop of the oil blend. Repeat three times—inhaling and exhaling nine times in total.

4 Put one drop of the oil blend on your thumb or index finger and then place the oil on the **Yintang** point, being careful not to let the oil touch your eyes or eyebrows. Gently massage nine small circles over the point.

5 Put one drop of the oil blend on your thumb or index finger and then place the oil on the Ren 17 point (**RN 17**). Gently massage the oil over the point with small circular motions.

6 Put one drop of the oil blend on the Pericardium 6 point (**PC 6**). Using your thumb or index finger, gently massage one small circle over the point.

7 Put one drop of the oil blend on your thumb or index finger and then place the oil on the Ren 6 point (**RN 6**). Gently massage nine small circles over the point.

8 Put one drop of the oil blend on your thumb or index finger and then place the oil on the Kidney 3 point (**KD 3**). Gently massage nine small circles over the point.

9 Use the palm inhalation technique to inhale one drop of the oil blend. Repeat three times—inhaling and exhaling nine times in total.

A BLEND TO BRING PEACE AND EMOTIONAL STABILITY

This treatment is beneficial if you feel unrooted, anxious, or nervous. It will help you feel more grounded and emotionally stable. The blend also nourishes the Blood.

You will need

5-ml blending bottle

Jojoba oil

2 drops vetiver oil

1 drop Roman chamomile oil

1 drop palmarosa oil

1. Fill the bottle with 1 teaspoon (5 ml) jojoba oil, then add the vetiver, Roman chamomile, and palmarosa oils and shake for a few moments.
2. Use the palm inhalation technique (see page 49) to inhale one drop of the oil blend.
3. Put one drop of the oil blend on your thumb or index finger and then place the oil on the Ren 17 point (**RN 17**). Gently massage nine small circles over the point.
4. Put one drop of the oil blend on your thumb or index finger and then place the oil on the Kidney 1 and/or the Kidney 3 point (**KD 1** and/or **KD 3**). Gently massage nine small circles over the point.
5. Put one drop of the oil blend on your thumb or index finger and then place the oil on the Spleen 6 point (**SP 6**). Gently massage nine small circles over the point.
6. Put one drop of the oil blend on your thumb or index finger and then place the oil on the Ren 4 point (**RN 4**). Gently massage nine small circles over the point.
7. Use the palm inhalation technique to inhale one drop of the oil blend. Repeat three times—inhaling and exhaling nine times in total.
8. Gently place the palm of your hand on or just below your navel. Hold it in place for at least three minutes.
9. Use the palm inhalation technique to inhale one drop of the oil blend.

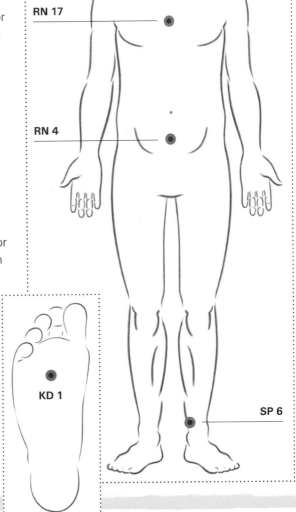

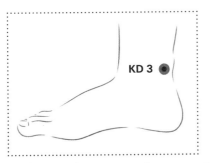

A BATH TO COOL HEART FIRE

This cooling bath will relax the nervous system and provide relief from the symptoms of emotional Fire, such as anger, frustration, and irritability. The ylang-ylang, palmarosa, and lavender oils all help to cool Fire and calm the Shen.

You will need

Small bowl

2 to 3 tablespoons (30 to 45 ml) liquid Castile soap (or you can use vegetable or jojoba oil)

2 drops ylang-ylang oil

1 drops palmarosa oil

1 drop lavender oil

1 Mix together the soap and essential oils in a small bowl.
2 Fill a bathtub with hot water, then add the soap mixture and swirl to mix well.
3 Get into the bath and soak in the water for about 20 minutes.

A BLEND TO AROUSE SEXUAL ENERGY

All three of the essential oils in this blend are aphrodisiacs that help to release inhibitions.

You will need

5-ml blending bottle

Jojoba oil

2 drops ylang-ylang oil

1 drop rose oil

1 drop jasmine oil

Warm moist compress (see page 52)

Towel

1 Fill the bottle with 1 teaspoon (5 ml) jojoba oil, then add the ylang-ylang, rose, and jasmine oils and shake for a few moments.
2 Place four drops of the oil blend in the palm of your hand, then add ½ teaspoon (2.5 ml) jojoba. Gently massage circles over your lower abdomen (just below your naval), adding another ½ teaspoon (2.5 ml) jojoba oil if necessary.
3 Lie down on your back. Place a warm moist compress on your lower abdomen, cover it with a dry towel, and leave it in place until the compress cools.

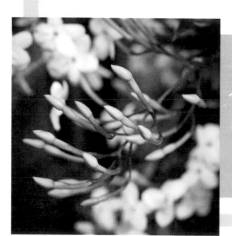

Chapter 5

Essential Oils to Help Increase Libido

- **Oils for men:** Cedarwood, cinnamon, Scots pine, rosemary, sandalwood, vetiver.
- **Oils for women:** Jasmine, rose, vetiver, ylang-ylang.

A BLEND FOR COOLING FIRE

German chamomile is associated with the Water element, and it can be used to cool the Fire element. This blend will help to relieve insomnia, anger, mood swings, and restlessness.

You will need

5-ml blending bottle

Jojoba oil

2 drops geranium oil

1 drop German chamomile oil

1 drop bergamot oil

1. Fill the bottle with 1 teaspoon (5 ml) jojoba oil, then add the geranium, German chamomile, and bergamot oils and shake for a few moments.
2. Use the palm inhalation technique (see page 49) to inhale one drop of the oil blend.
3. Put one drop of the oil blend on your thumb or index finger and then place the oil on the Du 14 point (**DU 14**). Gently massage three to nine small circles over the point.
4. Put one drop of the oil blend on the Pericardium 3 point (**PC 3**). Using your thumb or index finger, gently massage three to nine small circles over the point, then massage all the way down the Pericardium meridian to the end of the middle finger three to nine times.
5. Put one drop of the oil blend on your thumb or index finger and then place the oil on the Kidney 3 point (**KD 3**). Gently massage three to nine small circles over the point.
6. Use the palm inhalation technique to inhale one drop of the oil blend.

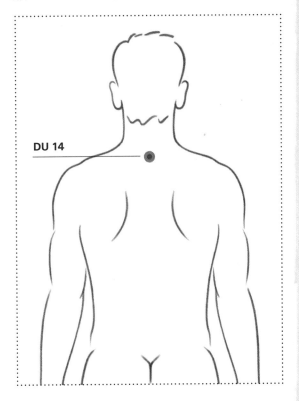

DU 14

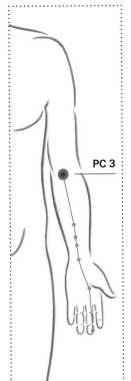

PC 3

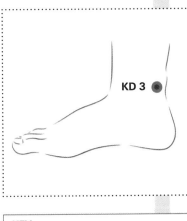

KD 3

KEY

—•— Pericardium meridian

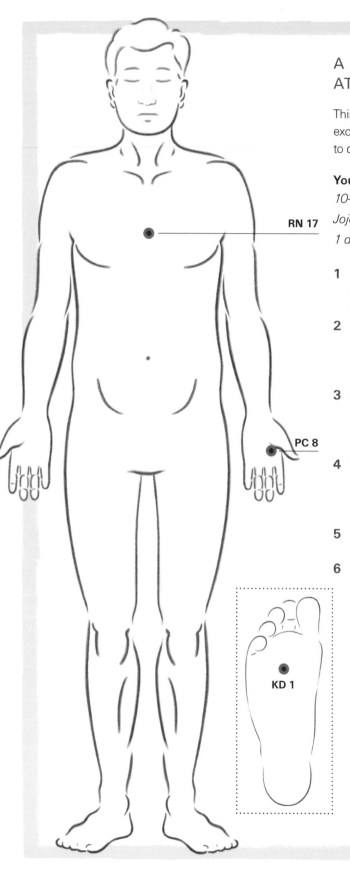

RN 17

PC 8

KD 1

A BLEND TO BRING EASE AT NIGHT

This blend will help alleviate restlessness and excitability in the evening by encouraging Yang to descend.

You will need

10-ml blending bottle

Jojoba oil

1 drop spikenard oil

1 Fill the bottle with 2 teaspoons (10 ml) jojoba oil, then add the spikenard oil and shake for a few moments.

2 Put one drop of the oil blend on your thumb or index finger and then place the oil on the Kidney 1 point (**KD 1**). Gently massage 9 to 27 small circles over the point.

3 Put one drop of the oil blend on your thumb or index finger and then place the oil on the Ren 17 point (**RN 17**). Gently massage three to nine small circles over the point.

4 Put one drop of the oil blend on the Pericardium 8 point (**PC 8**). Using your thumb or index finger, gently massage three to nine small circles over the point.

5 Use the palm inhalation technique (see page 49) to inhale one drop of the oil blend.

6 Gently place the palm of your hand on or just below your navel. Hold it in place for at least three minutes.

A BLEND TO STABILIZE THE SPIRIT

This treatment will calm the Shen.

You will need

5-ml blending bottle

Jojoba oil

1 drop bergamot oil (cools and calms the mind and cools Heart and Liver Fire)

1 drop lavender oil (cools Heart and Liver Fire and balances and uplifts Spikenard's downward nature)

1 drop geranium oil (cools Heart and Liver Fire and nourishes the Yin)

1 drop spikenard oil (cools Heart and Liver Fire and descends Qi)

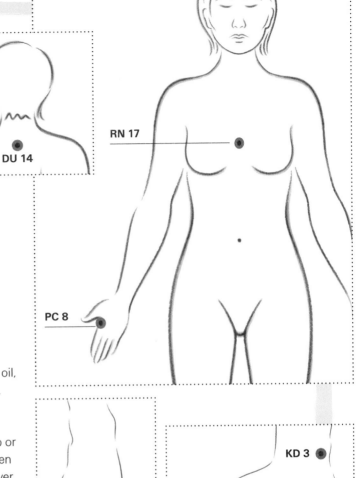

1 Fill the bottle with 1 teaspoon (5 ml) jojoba oil, then add the bergamot, lavender, geranium, and spikenard oils and shake for a few moments.

2 Put one drop of the oil blend on your thumb or index finger and then place the oil on the Ren 17 point (**RN 17**). Gently massage the oil over the point with small circular motions.

3 Put one drop of the oil blend on your thumb or index finger and then place the oil on the Du 14 point (**DU 14**). Gently massage the oil over the point with small circular motions.

4 Put one drop of the oil blend on your thumb or index finger and then place the oil on the Liver 3 point (**LV 3**). Gently massage the oil over the point with small circular motions.

5 Put one drop of the oil blend on your thumb or index finger and then place the oil on the Kidney 3 point (**KD 3**). Gently massage the oil over the point with circular motions.

6 Put one drop of the oil blend on the Pericardium 8 point (**PC 8**). Using your thumb or index finger, gently massage the oil over the point with small circular motions.

7 Use the palm inhalation technique (see page 49) to inhale one drop of the oil blend.

8 Gently place the palm of your hand on or just below your navel. Hold it in place for at least three minutes.

USING GINGER TO BUILD WILLPOWER

KEY
—•— Ren meridian

This treatment will help increase stamina and concentration.

You will need

5-ml blending bottle

Jojoba oil

3 drops ginger oil

1   Fill the bottle with 1 teaspoon (5 ml) jojoba oil, then add the ginger oil and shake for a few moments.
2   Use the palm inhalation technique (see page 49) to inhale one drop of the oil blend.
3   Put one drop of the oil blend on your thumb or index finger and then place the oil on the Ren 6 point (**RN 6**). As you inhale slowly and deeply, gently but firmly press into the point. Hold your breath for a couple of seconds, then exhale and release the point. Repeat nine times. Stroke upward to the Ren 17 point (**RN 17**) nine times. This will tonify the Qi.
4   Put one drop of the oil blend on your thumb or index finger and then place the oil on the Stomach 36 point (**ST 36**). As you inhale slowly and deeply, gently but firmly press into the point. Hold your breath for a couple of seconds, then exhale and release the point. Repeat nine times. This will tonify the Qi.
5   Put one drop of the oil blend on your thumb or index finger and then place the oil on the Kidney 3 point (**KD 3**). As you inhale slowly and deeply, gently but firmly press into the point. Hold your breath for a couple of seconds, then exhale and release the point. Repeat nine times. This will tonify the Qi and strengthen the will.

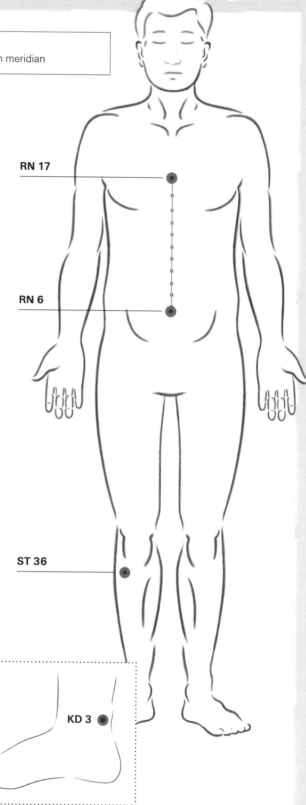

RN 17

RN 6

ST 36

KD 3

A PEACEFUL BATH

You will need
Small bowl

2 teapoons (10 ml) liquid Castile soap (or you can use vegetable or jojoba oil)

2 drops patchouli oil

1 drop geranium oil

1 drop frankincense oil

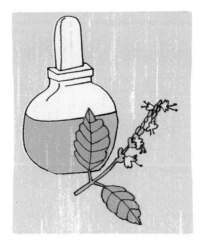

1   Mix together the soap and essential oils in a small bowl.
2   Fill a bathtub with hot water, then add the soap mixture and swirl to mix well.
3   Get into the bath and soak in the water for about 20 minutes.

A DIFFUSION TO INVIGORATE THE MIND AND IMPROVE FOCUS

You will need
Candle, mist, or electric diffuser

3 drops Eucalyptus radiata *oil*

2 drops peppermint oil

1 drop basil oil

1   Fill the diffuser with water and then add 1 drop each of the eucalyptus, peppermint, and basil oils.
2   Light the candle or turn on the diffuser. Wait a few minutes and then add the remaining drops of eucalyptus and peppermint oils if you like.

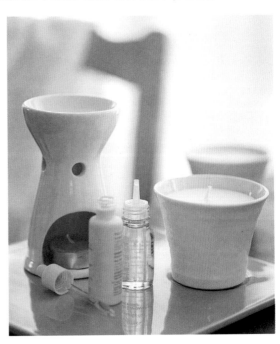

ACKNOWLEDGMENTS

First and foremost, I would like to thank my family and especially my mother—without their support this work would not be accomplished.

I would also like to thank my past students and teachers for giving me the platform to share information on aromatherapy and healing, and Tom Leung and Chava Quist at Kamwo Meridian Herbs for their ongoing support of my work (beyond aromatherapy) and the development of Meridian Biologix essential oils. I am especially thankful to Jeffery C. Yuen, for all his inspiration and teachings on Chinese medicine and aromatherapy. Thanks to Sandy Levine and all at the NY Open Center, to Joe Maggio (L. Ac) for his contribution to the chapter on meridians, and to Robert Tisserand and the Tisserand Institute for his ongoing research and teachings to advance the aromatherapy profession. Thanks to Raphael d'Angelo, a true healer, for his continued inspiration and guidance as my mentor in essential oils and aromatherapy, to Dr. Robert Fahey, for his continued inspiration and foresight, and to Dr. Peter Reznik, whose mentorship over the last 15 years has brought insight to the book, especially in the section on breath and healing.

I want to especially thank the publishing team—most notably Kristine Pidkameny, Carmel Edmonds, and Clare Churly for their time and effort in reading though the text and arranging it in such a way to make it usable and understandable for the readers. Also, thanks to the illustrators, Rosie Scott, Stephen Dew, and Cathy Brear, and designer, Emily Breen, for putting together such lovely charts and images of oils and meridians. Thank you.

NOTES

1. (p. 66), **2.** (p. 67), **3.** (p. 80), and **4.** (p.82) *Essential Oil Safety: A Guide for Health Care Professionals*, 2nd Edition, by Robert Tisserand and Rodney Young (Churchill Livingstone, 2013)